Peripheral T-cell Lymphomas

Edited by Pier Paolo Piccaluga

Published in London, United Kingdom

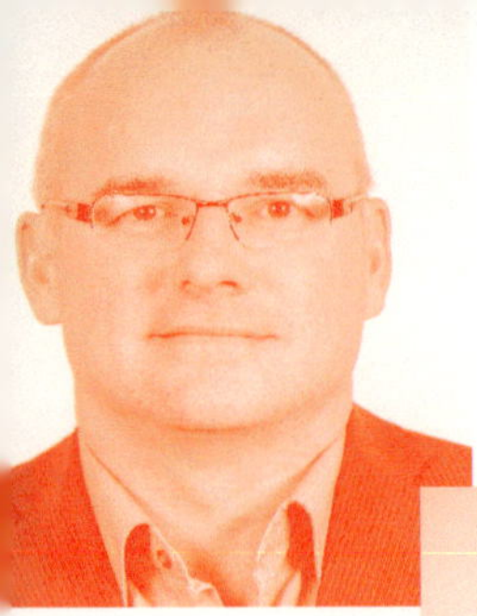
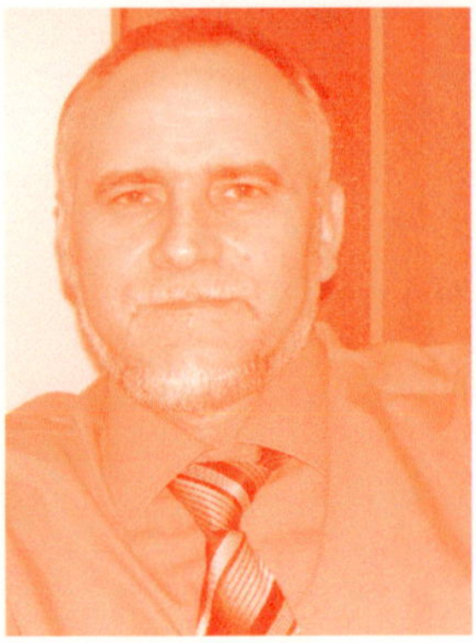
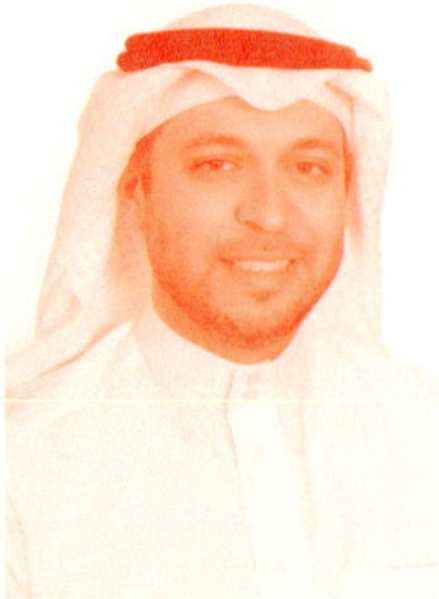
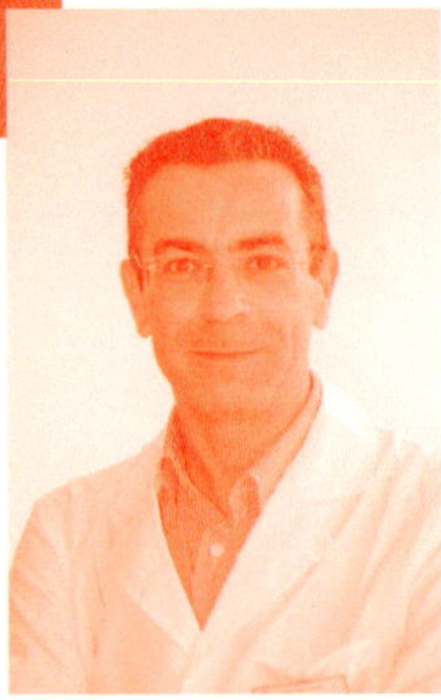
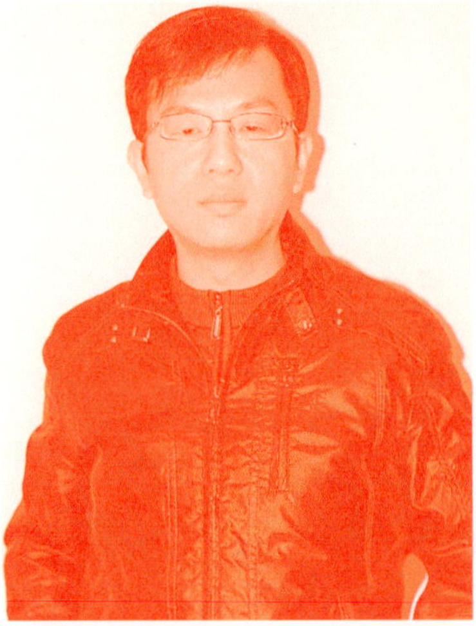
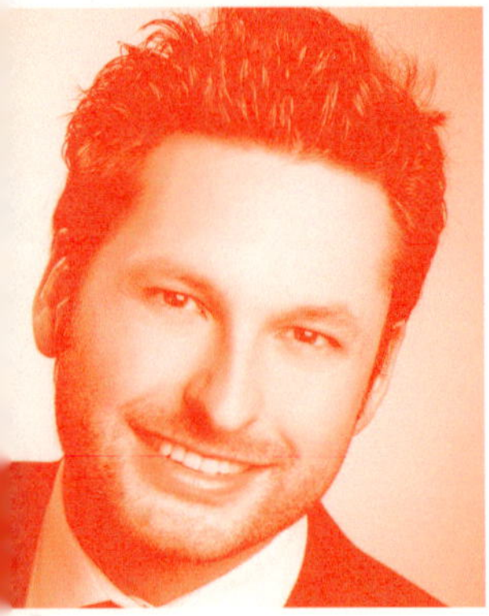
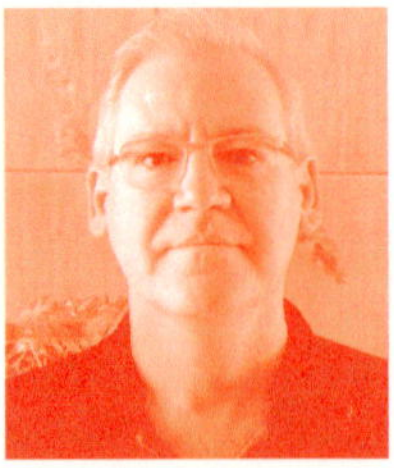

IntechOpen

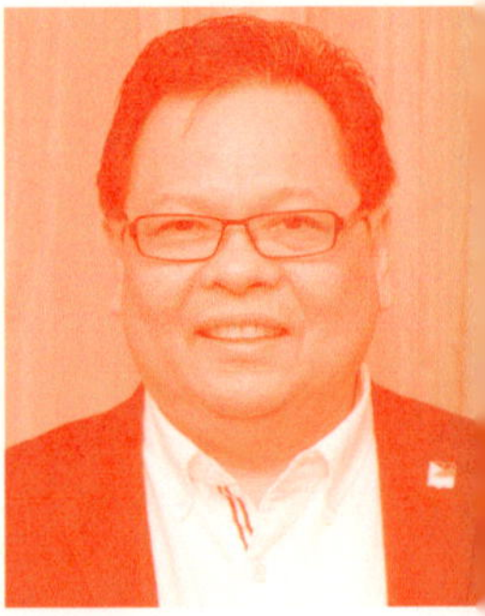
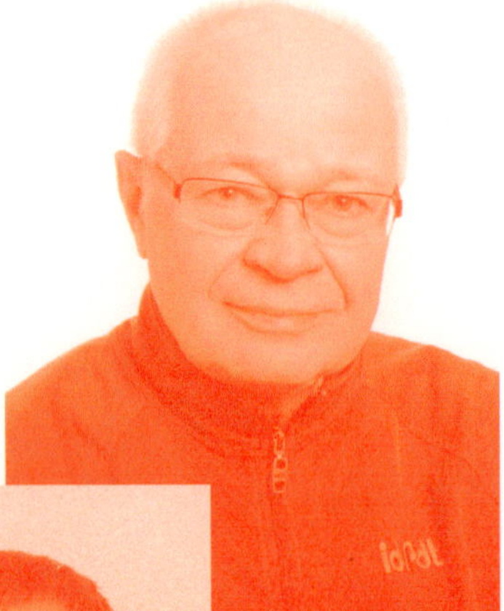
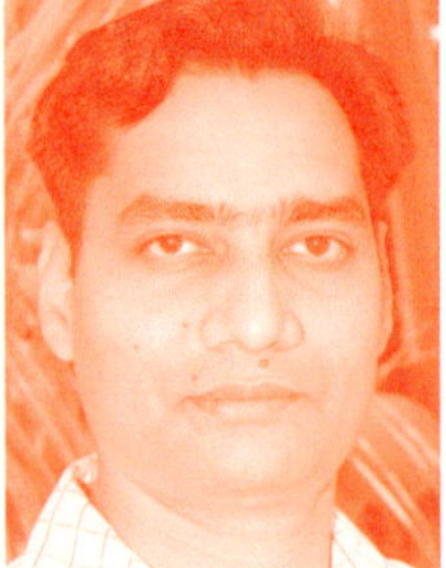
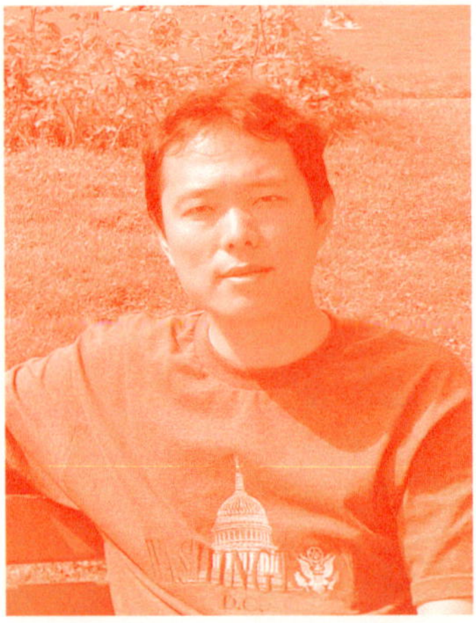
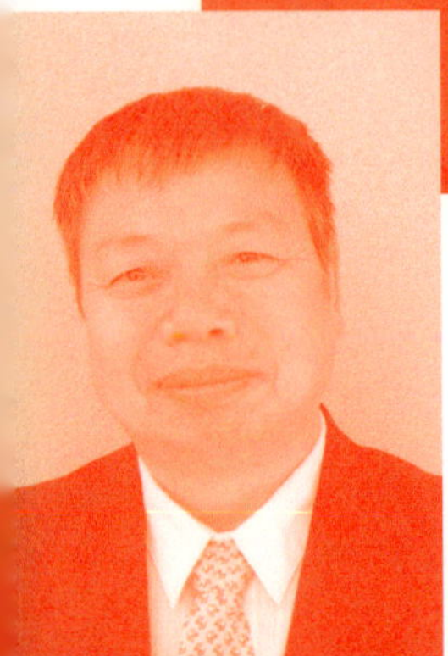
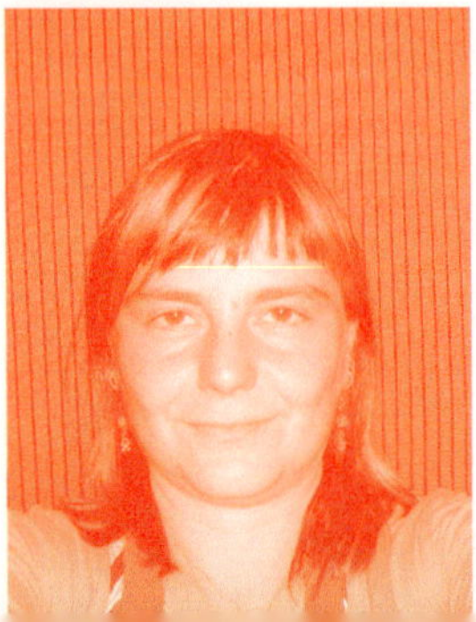

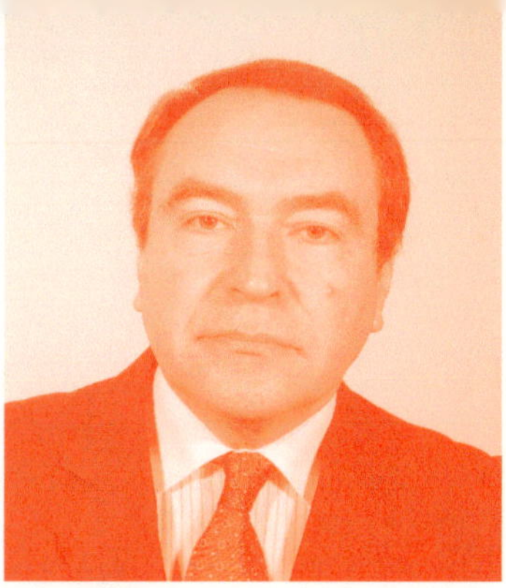
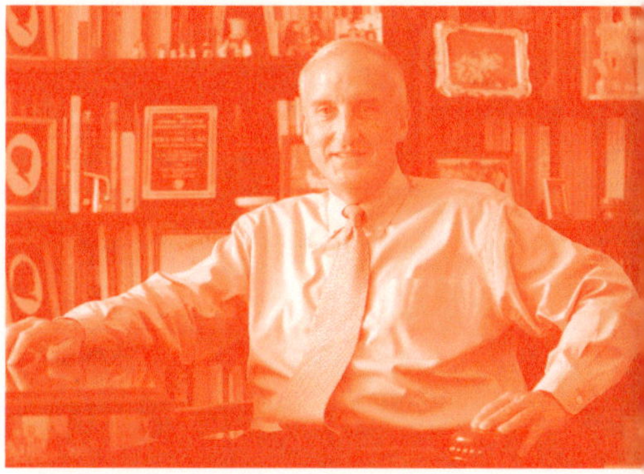
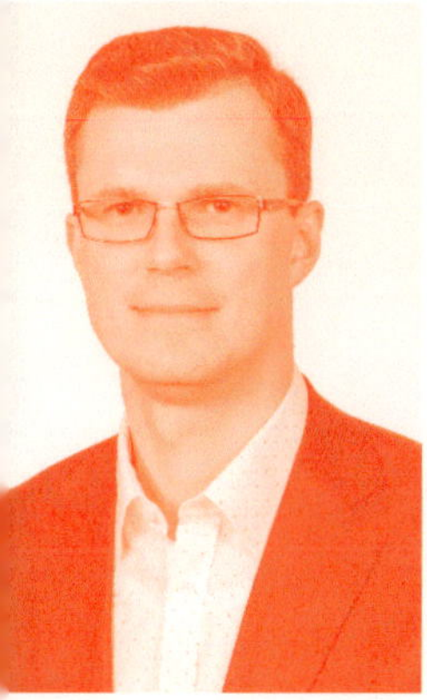
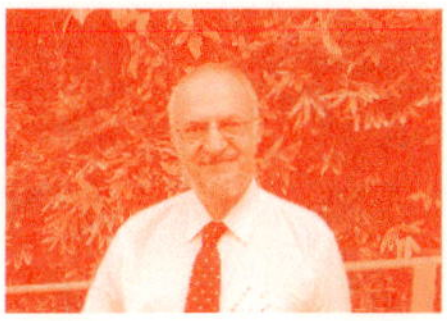
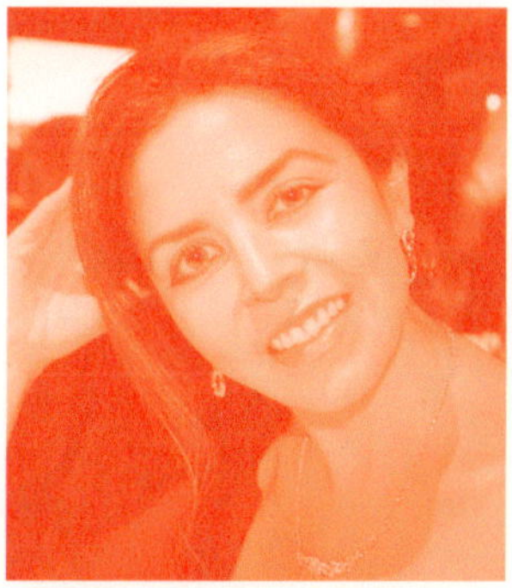

Supporting open minds since 2005

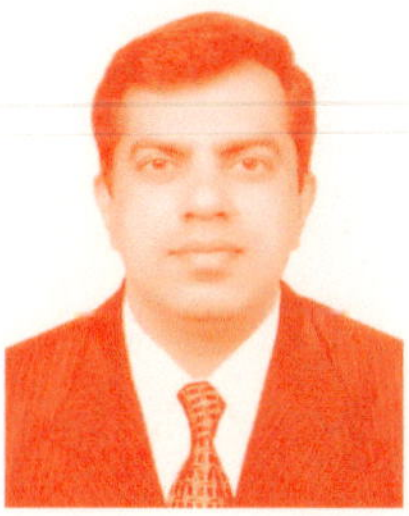
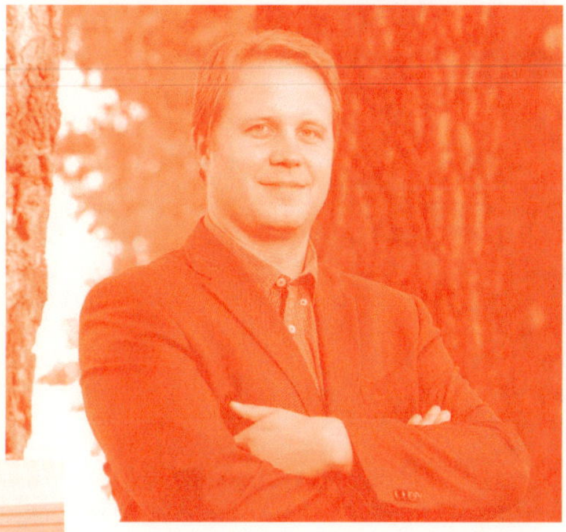
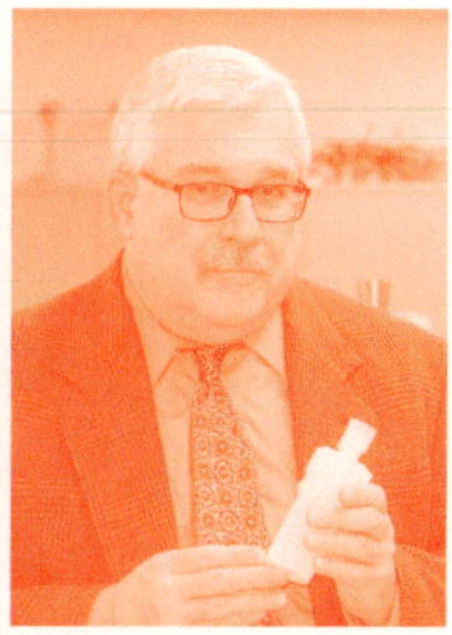
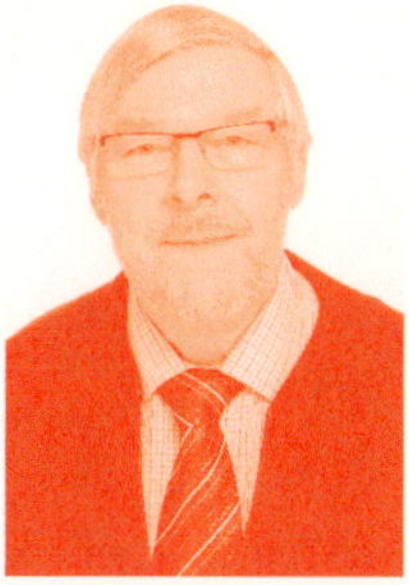
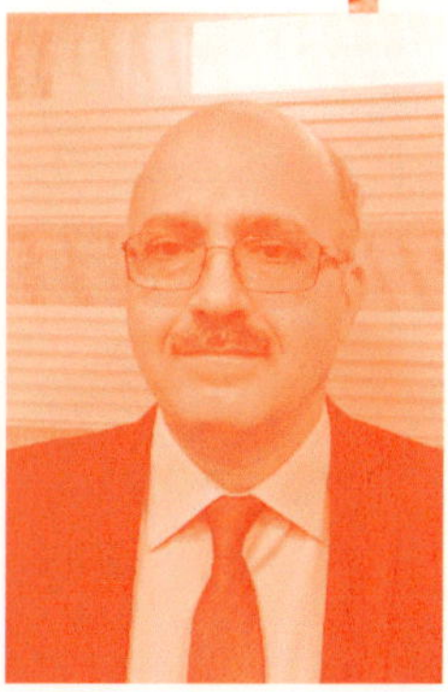
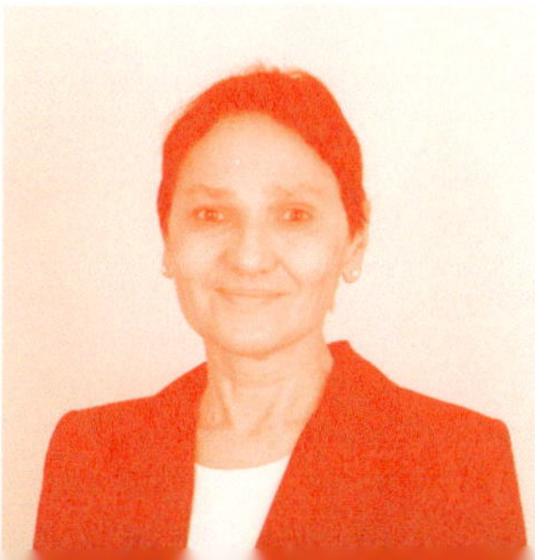
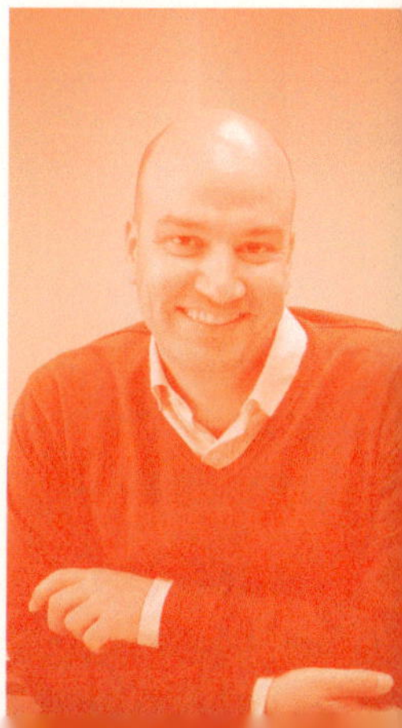

Peripheral T-cell Lymphomas
http://dx.doi.org/10.5772/intechopen.73947
Edited by Pier Paolo Piccaluga

Contributors
Suzanne Turner, Silvana Novelli, Soon Thye Lim, Nagavalli Somasundaram, Daruka Mahadevan, Pavan Tenneti, Lisa Davis, Jen Chin Wang, Preethi Ramachandran, Alok Aggarwal, Philipp Staber, Jennifer Amengual, Jacob Cogan, Pier Paolo Piccaluga

First published in London, United Kingdom, 2019 by IntechOpen
IntechOpen is the global imprint of INTECHOPEN LIMITED, registered in England and Wales, registration number: 11086078, The Shard, 25th floor, 32 London Bridge Street
London, SE19SG - United Kingdom
Printed in Croatia

British Library Cataloguing-in-Publication Data
A catalogue record for this book is available from the British Library

Additional hard and PDF copies can be obtained from orders@intechopen.com

Peripheral T-cell Lymphomas
Edited by Pier Paolo Piccaluga
p. cm.
Print ISBN 978-1-83881-225-6
Online ISBN 978-1-83881-226-3
eBook (PDF) ISBN 978-1-83881-227-0

For EU product safety concerns:
IN TECH d.o.o., Prolaz Marije Krucifikse Kozulić 3, 51000 Rijeka, Croatia, info@intechopen.com or visit our website at intechopen.com.

Meet the editor

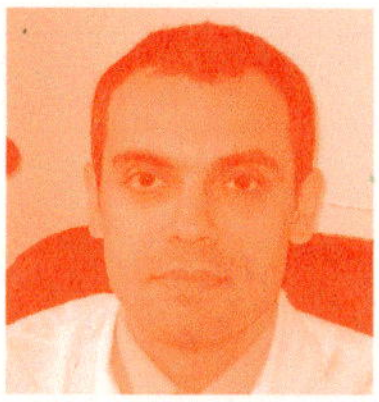

Pier Paolo Piccaluga is currently Associate Professor of Pathology at the Department of Experimental, Diagnostic and Specialty Medicine, Bologna University School of Medicine—Institute of Hematology and Medical Oncology, and has been responsible for many years for the Molecular Pathology Laboratory. In 2018 he was appointed for teaching at Queen Mary University of London (UK) and Jomo Kenyatta University of Agriculture and Technology, Nairobi (Kenya). He is the author of several international publications indexed in the Current Contents (215 publications quoted in PubMed, including *Nature Medicine*, *Journal of Clinical Investigation*, *Journal of Experimental Medicine*, *Journal of Clinical Oncology*, *Blood*, *Lancet Oncology*, and *Lancet Infectious Diseases*, with a total impact factor >1,000, a mean impact factor >6, and an H-index of 51 (ranked among the VIA-Academy Top Italian Scientists).

Contents

Preface

Tumors derived from T-lymphocytes are uncommon, representing 10% of lymphoid malignancies overall and encompassing several extremely rare different entities. However, they represent an important diagnostic and therapeutic challenge. In fact, on the one hand, their rarity, heterogeneity, as well as the lack of specific diagnostic markers make their diagnosis quite difficult. Indeed, large studies performed in Europe and the United States showed that up to 30% of cases are misdiagnosed. On the other hand, largely due to their rarity, the currently used therapeutic schemes are basically derived from those adopted for B-cell malignancies and appear definitely unsatisfactory. Only recently have specific clinical trials been dedicated to T-cell lymphomas, leading to the approval of a few new drugs for second-line treatments. Hopefully, currently ongoing trials will be able to show some benefit when such new drugs are included in first-line approaches as well.

In this book, a brief overview on the most updated World Health Organization (WHO) classification and the general features of peripheral T-cell lymphomas (PTCLs) is first provided. Thereafter, a few entities have been described in more detail and, eventually, new concepts of personalized targeted treatments are listed and discussed. A particular emphasis has been given to anaplastic large cell lymphomas, the classification of which has been significantly modified in the new WHO blue book, now including anaplastic lymphoma kinase-positive and -negative forms, as well as the cutaneous and breast implant-associated types. Similarly, non-cutaneous and gamma-delta T-cell lymphomas has been described according to their new classification. In all sections and chapters, the role of molecular genetics has been considered, highlighting its role in the development of novel classification as well as of new, more rational targeted approaches. In fact, the better understanding of PTCL pathophysiology, largely based on gene expression profiling and next-generation sequencing studies, had a pivotal role in the definition of novel targets for more effective therapies. As prototypic examples of this process, therapies targeting the epigenetic machinery as well as Aurora kinase inhibitors have been deeply described. It should not be forgotten, nonetheless, that the prognosis of PTCL patients is still generally dismal and extensive basic and clinical research have to be carried out in the future to improve the present scenario.

The book is intended for all health professionals, particularly for those involved in the diagnosis and treatment of oncological diseases, as well as medical students and fellows.

As editor, I am indeed grateful to IntechOpen, and especially Ms. Sara Debeuc, for help and support, as well as to all the authors contributing to this book.

Pier Paolo Piccaluga, MD, PhD
Professor,
Institute of Hematology and Medical Oncology,
Department of Experimental, Diagnostic and Specialty Medicine,
Bologna University School of Medicine,
Bologna, Italy

Chapter 1

Introductory Chapter: Updates and New Insights from WHO 2017 Peripheral T-Cell Lymphoma Classification

Pier Paolo Piccaluga

1. Introduction

Peripheral T-cell lymphomas (PTCLs) are relatively rare disorders, representing around 10% of all lymphomas worldwide; however, they are relatively common in specific geographic areas, including Asia, the Caribbean basin, and scattered areas in Europe where HTVL1 is endemic.

In the latest edition of the World Health Organisation (WHO) Classification of Tumours of Haematopoietic and Lymphoid Tissues, edited in 2017, nodal, extra nodal and leukaemia forms are listed. Specifically, as many as 31 entities are listed among PTCLs [1]. Compared with the previous edition, in the current classification, a few but quite relevant novelties have been introduced. Generally speaking, as already observed for B-cell derived malignancies, recent discoveries from molecular genetic studies led to a better definition of certain entities and clearly defined a pivotal role for cellular derivation in tumour classification. In the following, the main updates concerning non-cutaneous PTCLs will be briefly discussed.

2. T-follicular helper cell-related lymphomas

Among nodal PTCLs, that overall constitute the majority of PTCL cases, a new subgroups has been defined based on the corresponding to a specific cellular counterpart, namely the T-follicular helper (TFH) lymphocytes. The latter is physiologically represented within germinal centres of secondary follicles, providing costimulatory signalling to B-lymphocytes through many different singling pathways [2]. These cells, at immunophenotyping, are characterised by the expression of selected markers, including BCL6, SAP, ICOS, CXCL13 and CD10. Consistently, tutors derived from TFH cells express these molecules. However, likely due to the aberrancy in phenotype, which is typical of PTCLS [3], some of them may lack in a single case. Therefore, an extended panel should be tested to confirm the diagnosis. On the other hand, since non-TFH-derived PTCLs may express one of these markers, it is recommended to detect positive staining for at least two (better would be three) of them to claim a TFH derivation [4]. TFH-related PTCLs currently include three main nodal PTCL types, namely angioimmunoblastic T-cell lymphoma (AITL, the commonest PTCL in northern Europe), follicular T-cell lymphoma (FTCL, formerly accounted among PTCLS not otherwise specified/NOS), and PTCL/NOS not fulfilling the diagnostic criteria for the previous tutors but showing

IntechOpen

a clear TFH-phenotype. Such cases were characterised and associated to TFH-lymphocyte at both transcriptional and protein level [5–7].

Beside the cell of origin, *per se* relevant criteria for tumour classification, TFH-related PTCLs also share, at least for a certain extent, the genetic background and, therefore, the molecular pathogenesis. Particularly, genes controlling epigenetic regulation of gene expression as well as gene involved in T-cell receptor (TCR) signalling appeared to be more commonly deregulated [8, 9]. The presence of *TET2, IDH2* and *DNMT3A/B* somatic mutations is detected in about 20–80% of cases [10, 11]. Intriguingly, it was recently shown that treatment with 5-azacytidine, a well-known demethylating agent, currently approved for acute myeloid leukaemia therapy, was strikingly effective in patients affected by TFH-PTCL, with sustained clinical responses observed in previously relapsed/refractory cases [12]. Second, mutations affecting *RHOA* were observed in up to 70% of AITL cases and in a variable percentage of other PTCLs [9, 11]. By deregulating the RHOA GTPase protein, the TCR signalling is eventually affected. Similar effects are determined by *VAV1* rearrangements that are mutually exclusive with *RHOA* mutations. Less frequently, other genetic events can inter with TCR singling, including *PLCG1* (14%), *CD28* (9–11%) and *FYN* (3–4%) [8].

Finally, ITK/SYK rearrangements, due to the t(5;9) translocation, are quite common in FTCL, being only occasionally recorded in AITL.

Therapeutic strategies designed against aberrant TCR are currently under investigation.

3. Extra-nodal, non-cutaneous PTCL

As far as this category of PTCLs is concerned, the main novelties regard anaplastic large cell lymphomas (ALCLs) and intestinal PTCLs.

Among ALCLs, first of all, ALCL ALK-negative has been regarded as an independent entity, mainly based on gene expression data [13-15] and more recent genetic data acquired through next generation sequencing [16]. In fact, ALCL ALK-negative was shown to have a global gene expression profile (GEP) different from other PTCLs and specially PTCL/NOS, carrying recurrent genetic rearrangements eventually leading to STAT3 activation [16]. Noteworthy, this finding provides the molecular basis for the similarities between ALCL ALK-positive and negative, since STAT3 is the main downstream of ALK as well.

Second, a new provisional entity has been introduced, the breast-implant-associated (BI) ALCL. This tumour, although very uncommon, solicited great attention for the social impact. In fact, it selectively arises in patients who received a breast implant after oncologic or simply aesthetic surgery. The tumour can present as wither a serum (i.e. with malignant cells floating in a serous fluid around the capsule) or as tumbrel mass, the latter cases being more aggressive. Of note, recent GEP studies indicated that BI-ALCL is distinct from ALK-positive and negative cases, but presents with the same typical features including STAT3 activation and TCR singling downregulation [17]. The genetic background of the disease needs, however, to be fully elucidated.

As far as intestinal PTCLs are concerned, it has become apparent that the two subtypes formerly designated as variants of enteropathy-associated T-cell lymphoma (EATL) are distinct [18–20]. Type I EATL, now designated as EATL, is closely related to coeliac disease and is mainly encountered in people from the northern part of Europe. Type II EATL, now designated as *monomorphic epitheliotropic intestinal T-cell lymphoma (MEITL)*, shows no link with coeliac disease and appears relatively more common in Hispanic and Asian populations. Genetically, gains in chromosome 8q24 involving MYC are seen in a high proportion of cases of MEITL but not EATL. On the clinical ground, both forms of intestinal T-cell lymphoma are aggressive and almost always occur in adults [18].

Overall, a new road towards molecular classification and possibly more targeted therapy has been initiated for PTCLs, as it happened for acute leukemias and B-cell lymphomas in the last decade. Despite the large amount of still unsolved issues, hopefully, this will be translated soon into significant benefit for patients and communities.

Author details

Pier Paolo Piccaluga[1,2,3]

1 Department of Experimental, Diagnostic and Specialty Medicine, Institute of Hematology and Medical Oncology "L&A Seràgnoli", Bologna University School of Medicine, Bologna, Italy

2 Euro-Mediterranean Institute of Science and Technology (IEMEST), Palermo, Italy

3 Department of Pathology, Jomo Kenyatta University of Agriculture and Technology, Nairobi, Kenya

*Address all correspondence to: pierpaolo.piccaluga@unibo.it

References

[1] Swerdlow SH, Campo E, Harris NL, Jaffe ES, Pileri SA, Stein H, Thiele J. WHO Classification of tumors of hematopoietic and lymphoid tissues. 5th ed. Vol. 1. Lyon: IARC; 2017

[2] CG1 V, Linterman MA, Yu D, MacLennan IC. Follicular helper T cells. Annual Review of Immunology. 2016;**34**:335-368

[3] Went P, Agostinelli C, Gallamini A. Marker expression in peripheral T-cell lymphoma: A proposed clinical-pathologic prognostic score. Journal of Clinical Oncology. 2006;**24**(16):2472-2479

[4] Dogan A, Gaulard P, Jaffe ES. Angioimmunoblastic T-cell lymphoma and other nodal lymphomas of T follicular helper cell origin. In: WHO Classification of tumors of hematopoietic and lymphoid tissues. 5th ed. Vol. 1. Lyon: IARC; 2017. pp. 407-412

[5] Rudiger T, Geissinger E, Muller-Hermelink HK. 'Normal counterparts' of nodal peripheral T-cell lymphoma. Hematological Oncology. 2006;**24**(4):175-180

[6] de Leval L, Rickman DS, Thielen C, et al. The gene expression profile of nodal peripheral T-cell lymphoma demonstrates a molecular link between angioimmunoblastic T-cell lymphoma (AITL) and follicular helper T (TFH) cells. Blood. 2007;**109**(11):4952-4963

[7] Piccaluga PP, Agostinelli C, Califano A, et al. Gene expression analysis of angioimmunoblastic lymphoma indicates derivation from T follicular helper cells and vascular endothelial growth factor deregulation. Cancer Research. 2007;**67**(22):10703-10710

[8] Vallois D, Dobay MP, Morin RD, et al. Activating mutations in genes related to TCR signaling in angioimmunoblastic and other follicular helper T-cell-derived lymphomas. Blood. 2016;**128**(11):1490-1502

[9] Palomero T, Couronne L, Khiabanian H, et al. Recurrent mutations in epigenetic regulators, RHOA and FYN kinase in peripheral T cell lymphomas. Nature Genetics. 2014;**46**(2):166-170

[10] Lemonnier F, Couronne L, Parrens M, et al. Recurrent TET2 mutations in peripheral T-cell lymphomas correlate with TFH-like features and adverse clinical parameters. Blood. 2012;**120**(7):1466-1469

[11] Odejide O, Weigert O, Lane AA. A targeted mutational landscape of angioimmunoblastic T-cell lymphoma. Blood. 2014;**123**(9):1293-1296

[12] Lemonnier F, Dupuis J, Sujobert P. Treatment with 5-azacytidine induces a sustained response in patients with angioimmunoblastic T-cell lymphoma. Blood. 2018;**132**(21):2305-2309

[13] Piccaluga PP, Agostinelli C, Califano A, et al. Gene expression analysis of peripheral T cell lymphoma, unspecified, reveals distinct profiles and new potential therapeutic targets. The Journal of Clinical Investigation. 2007;**117**(3):823-834

[14] Piva R, Agnelli L, Pellegrino E. Gene expression profiling uncovers molecular classifiers for the recognition of anaplastic large-cell lymphoma within peripheral T-cell neoplasms. Journal of Clinical Oncology. 2010;**28**(9):1583-1590

[15] Iqbal J, Weisenburger DD, Greiner TC, et al. Molecular signatures to improve diagnosis in peripheral T-cell lymphoma and prognostication in angioimmunoblastic T-cell lymphoma. Blood. 2010;**115**(5):11

[16] Crescenzo R, Abate F, Lasorsa E. Convergent mutations and kinase

fusions lead to oncogenic STAT3 activation in anaplastic large cell lymphoma. Cancer Cell. 2015;**27**(4):516-532

[17] Di Napoli A, De Cecco L, Piccaluga PP. Transcriptional analysis distinguishes breast implant-associated anaplastic large cell lymphoma from other peripheral T-cell lymphomas. Modern Pathology. 2019;**32**(2):216-230

[18] Jaffe ES, Chott A, Ott G. Intestinal T-cell lymphoma. In: WHO Classification of tumors of hematopoietic and lymphoid tissues. 5th ed. Vol. 1. Lyon: IARC; 2017. pp. 372-380

[19] Attygalle AD, Cabegadas J, Gaulard P, et al. Peripheral T-cell and NK-cell lymphomas and their mimics; taking a step forward - report on the lymphoma workshop of the XVIth meeting of the European Association for Haematopathology and the Society for Hematopathology. Histopathology. 2014;**64**:171-199

[20] Swerdlow SH, Jaffe ES, Brousset P, et al. Cytotoxic T-cell and NK-cell lympho mas: Current questions and controversies. The American Journal of Surgical Pathology. 2014;**38**:e60-e71

Chapter 2

Overview of T-cell Lymphomas

Nagavalli Somasundaram and Soon Thye Lim

Abstract

T-cell lymphomas are a mixed bag of diseases with a similar origin but diverse in biology and behavior. This review aims to highlight the key changes to the WHO classification and summarize the therapeutic paradigm as of the time of writing in November 2018.

Keywords: T-cell lymphoma, transplant

1. Introduction

T- and natural killer (NK)-cell lymphomas are a heterogeneous group of lymphoproliferative diseases that represent 10–15% of non-Hodgkin lymphomas (NHL). T-cell lymphomas in general have worse outcomes as compared to their B-cell counterparts. Over recent years, the understanding of the different subtypes of T-cell lymphoma has led to advances in management.

2. Background

2.1 WHO classification

T- and NK-cell lymphomas can be subclassified according to nodal, extranodal, cutaneous, or leukemic subtypes based on the 2008 World Health Organization (WHO) classification of lymphoid malignancies (**Table 1**) [1]. The 2016 update of the WHO classification saw the addition of three provisional entities and changes in designation to five entities, reflecting the advancements in the understanding of this group of diseases [2, 3]. The major changes are highlighted below.

The update in the classification saw follicular T-cell lymphoma coming under the umbrella of angioimmunoblastic T-cell lymphoma (AITL), given the common genetic mutations such as *TET2*, *IDH2*, *DNMT3A*, *RHOA*, and *CD28* and fusions such as *ITK-SYK* and *CTLA4-CD28* nodal peripheral T-cell lymphoma (PTCL), previously classified under peripheral T-cell lymphoma, not otherwise specified (PTCL NOS) was reclassified under the AITL classification given the similar genetic landscape.

The diagnosis of PTCL NOS is made when a lymphoproliferative disorder is of the T-cell lineage without any distinctive features that fit into the subtypes. Two distinct molecular subgroups have been identified in PTCL NOS with differing clinical outcomes and prognosis. High expression of transcription factor *GATA3* was associated with worse clinical outcomes, while TBX2 expression enriched by IFNgamma and NfKB pathways was associated with better survival. These findings provide insight into a disease which has been a diagnosis of exclusion, with poor clinical outcomes and minimal advances in treatment.

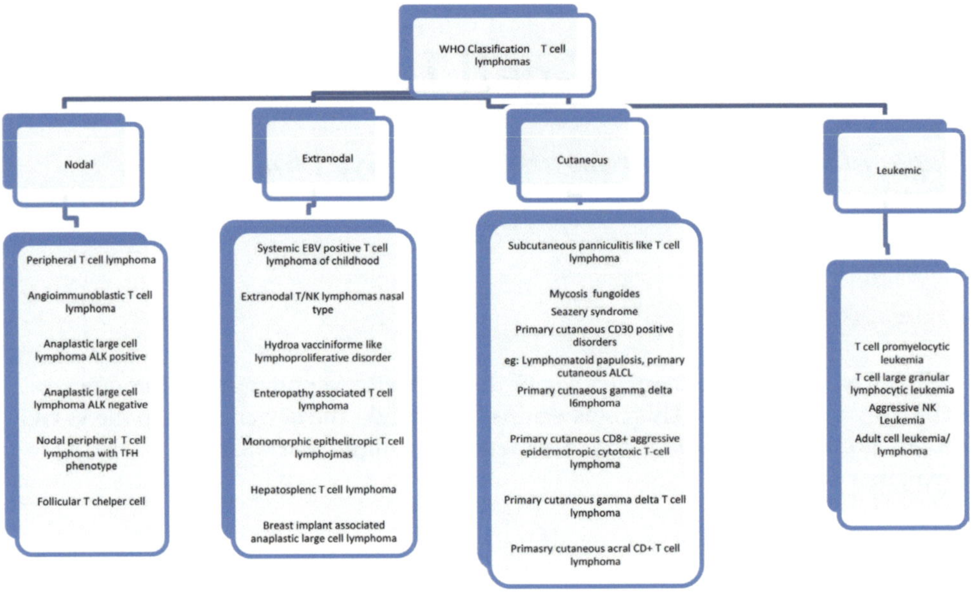

Table 1.
Classification of T-cell lymphoma.

The ALK-negative subtype of anaplastic large cell lymphoma (ALCL) has been identified as a distinct entity. The expression of *TNFRSF8*, *BATF*, and *TMOD1* differentiates ALK-negative ALCL from PTCL NOS. ALK-negative ALCL is a heterogeneous disease with a third harboring *DUSP22* rearrangement and another 8% having *TP63* rearrangements. The former has a 90% 5-year overall survival (OS) rate, mirroring the outcomes of its ALK-positive ALCL counterpart, while the latter is associated with a 5-year OS rate of 17%. The subset of ALK-negative ALCL which does not carry both the rearrangements has outcomes straddling in between these two extremes.

Breast implant-associated ALCL has been recognized as a provisional new entity—this is a unique variant in that the lymphomatous cells are confined to the seroma fluid surrounding the implant without capsular invasion. As such, surgical removal of the implant including the capsule is often curative, with systemic therapy being rarely indicated.

The 2008 classification included enteropathy-associated T-cell lymphoma (EATL) types 1 and 2 as part of the intestinal T-cell lymphoma spectrum. In the latest revision, this has been amended to EATL and monomorphic epitheliotropic intestinal T-cell lymphoma (MEITL). EATL is a condition linked to coeliac disease and is more common among northern Europeans. MEITL, on the other hand, is a disease of Asians and Hispanics with no associations with coeliac disease. At a molecular level, EATL is predominantly characterized by T-cell alpha/beta receptor expression, while MEITL has predominantly T-cell gamma/delta receptors being expressed. The nuclear expression of megakaryocyte-associated tyrosine kinase, MYC amplification, and alterations in SETD2 and JAK STAT pathways are other genetic events characteristic of MEITL [4].

2.2 Epidemiology

PTCL NOS forms about 25% of T-cell lymphomas, followed by angioimmunoblastic T-cell lymphomas (18%), NK-/T-cell lymphomas (NKTL—10%), and adult T leukemia/lymphoma (9%) [5]. Geographic variation in the various subtypes of T-cell lymphoma has been reported. The international T-cell lymphoma study reported rates of PTCL and NKTL to be 5–10% in Western countries and 10–20% in Asian countries. However, Au et al., in a study of 148 patients, reported similar frequencies of T-cell lymphomas in the Western and Asian populations [6]. This was supported by another study analyzing the differences between PTCL and NKTL [7]. The perceived difference in the disparate frequencies of these diseases may have been contributed by a higher incidence of NKTL and adult T-cell lymphoma/leukemia (ATLL) in the Asian population.

3. Clinical aspects

3.1 Clinical characteristics

PTCL NOS is a disease of older adults with a median age of 60. It often presents at advanced stages with both nodal and extranodal sites of disease, with cutaneous and bone marrow involvement being the most common extranodal sites [5, 8].

Angioimmunoblastic T-cell lymphoma (AITL) is a multifaceted disease with a spectrum of clinical presentations, from fairly indolent disease to aggressive presentations. Similar to PTCL NOS, it is also a disease of older adults. Patients often present in advanced stages with B symptoms being the most common clinical manifestation. Bone marrow, liver, spleen, and skin involvements are common in this disease [9]. Immune-related phenomena such as hemolytic anemia, hypergammaglobulinemia, and positive Coombs test are associated with AITL [10].

Anaplastic large cell lymphomas (ALCL) are CD30-positive T-cell lymphoproliferative disorders with about half having ALK gene rearrangement (ALK + ALCL). The ALK-positive variant occurs in young adults with a median age of 30, while the ALK-negative ALCL is a disease of older adults. Systemic ALCLs have a varying clinical course and prognosis compared to their cutaneous counterparts, with the latter having an indolent course of disease with long-term survival in the range of 85–95% [11]. Central nervous system involvement is seen more commonly in ALCL than other T-cell lymphoma subtypes.

Extranodal NK-/T-cell lymphoma, nasal type, and aggressive NK-cell leukemia are the different subtypes of NKTL. NKTL commonly involves the nasal cavity and the upper aerodigestive tract. While localized disease is often treated with curative intent, advanced disease is invariably fatal. A small proportion of advanced NKTL patients can present with hemophagocytic syndrome resulting in high fevers, cytopenias, coagulopathy, abnormal liver function tests, and very high ferritin levels.

Adult T-cell leukemia/lymphoma is a disease of adolescents and young adults. Extensive marrow involvement defines the leukemic variant of this disease, while the lymphoma variant has less than 20% marrow involvement. This is a highly aggressive disease with common presentations including bulky mediastinal masses or nodal disease [12].

Cutaneous T-cell lymphoma (CTCL) is a heterogeneous group of disease, with mycosis fungoides and Sezary syndrome being the most common subtypes. The incidence of the various subtypes often increases with age [13]. CTCLs are generally indolent diseases, but large cell transformation is generally associated with poor outcomes [14].

3.2 Workup and diagnosis

Workup of T-cell lymphomas involves a complete history and physical examination followed by routine laboratory evaluation including full blood count, assessment of end-organ function, lactate dehydrogenase levels, and screening for human immunodeficiency virus, hepatitis B and C. Epstein-Barr virus (EBV) DNA testing using EBV PCR can be considered in EBV-positive tumors. Plasma EBV detection can serve as a marker to monitor disease response and as a prognostic factor in these settings [15]. Staging evaluations include radiological imaging and bone marrow biopsy [18]. Fluorodeoxyglucose positron emission tomography combined with computer tomography (PET CT) is gaining an increasing role in the initial staging of T-cell lymphomas. Given the high propensity for extranodal involvement, some of which (e.g., cutaneous involvement) may not be well demarcated on CT, PET CT may be useful as an initial staging modality. A retrospective study demonstrated that almost a third of the patients in the study had additional sites of disease picked up on PET CT beyond conventional CT imaging [16]. In NKTL, PET CT has been established as a standard staging investigation given its high sensitivity and specificity [17].

The diagnosis of T-cell lymphomas should ideally be made by a hematopathologist. An excisional biopsy is recommended whenever possible in order to ensure availability of adequate tissue sample for histopathological analysis. According to the WHO classification in 2008, the diagnosis of PTCL requires the integration of clinical, pathological, immunohistochemical, and molecular findings.

4. Management

At present there is no standard of care available for management of T-cell lymphoma as a result of paucity of randomized controlled phase 3 trials. Anthracycline-based regimens such as cyclophosphamide, vincristine, doxorubicin, and prednisolone (CHOP) have been the backbone of treatment for many decades for most subtypes of T-cell lymphomas, with the exception of NKTL. The international T-cell lymphoma project, with a predominant European and Asian population, demonstrated that there was no survival benefit seen with an anthracycline-based regimen for PTCL NOS and AITL [5]. A subsequent retrospective study in a north American population showed 25 months improvement in survival with the use of an anthracycline-based regimen, even after controlling for confounding factors [18]. Nevertheless, unlike the B-cell counterparts, T-cell lymphomas in general have a poorer outcome, with 5-year overall survival being about 30%.

In NKTL, anthracycline-based regimens were abandoned early on with the discovery that NK cells have a high expression of multidrug-resistant P-glycoprotein. Hence, drugs that are transported by P-glycoproteins such as cyclophosphamide and doxorubicin become ineffective [19]. L-asparaginase is an enzyme that induces cytotoxicity to lymphoma/leukemic cells by catalyzing the hydrolysis of L-asparagine, thereby resulting in its depletion. This drug has been demonstrated to have significant in vitro activity against NK cells [20] and hence has been incorporated into the treatment regimens. Hence, in advanced NKTL, L-asparaginase-based multiagent chemotherapy has been adopted as first-line treatment.

4.1 Strategies to improve first-line treatment

4.1.1 Intensive chemotherapy

Multiple strategies have been explored in order to overcome the poor treatment outcomes in T-cell lymphomas. A retrospective study by MD Anderson group demonstrated that more intensive regimens such as HyperCVAD and HyperCHOP did not fare better than conventional CHOP in non-ALCL T-cell lymphomas. The 3-year overall survival was 49% in the intensive treatment group as compared to 43% in the CHOP group, and this was not statistically significant [21].

The GOELAMS-LTP95 was a phase 3 randomized trial that compared alternating cycles of VIP and rABVD (etoposide, ifosfamide, cisplatin—VIP; reinforced adriamycin, bleomycin, vinblastine, dacarbazine—rABVD) against CHOP for non-cutaneous T-cell lymphomas. There was no significant difference in the 2-year event-free survival, which was the primary endpoint of the study [22].

Gemcitabine, cisplatin, and methylprednisolone were compared to CHOP in the treatment of T-cell lymphomas in the first-line setting in a phase 2 trial. This CHEMO-T trial did not show any improvements in complete response rates, progression-free or overall survival rates between four cycles of GEM-P and six cycles of CHOP [23].

Hence, intensifying first-line chemotherapy as a strategy has not improved outcomes in T-cell lymphomas.

4.1.2 Addition of etoposide

The NHL B1 and B2 studies were designed to answer the questions of whether addition of etoposide to CHOP or increasing dose intensity of CHOP will improve outcomes in patients with aggressive lymphomas. T-cell lymphoma patients formed 13.7 and 5.8% of the study populations in NHL B1 [24] and B2 [25] studies, respectively. In young patients, addition of etoposide improved event-free survival by about 10%, but this did not translate into improvement in overall survival. In older patients, the addition of etoposide did not improve progression-free or overall survival compared to CHOP 14 which became the German standard of care following the NHL B2 trial.

A retrospective review of patients treated in trials designed by the German non-Hodgkin lymphoma study group showed an improvement in 3-year event-free survival (EFS) from 51 to 75.1% ($p = 0.03$). However, this difference in EFS was predominantly contributed by the ALK-positive ALCL—the EFS in this subgroup improved markedly from 57.1 to 91.2% with the addition of etoposide. The difference in EFS was no longer statistically significant when this group was removed from the analysis [26].

Similar results were noted in a retrospective study by a Swedish group which analyzed 755 patients with T-cell lymphoma. Improvement in EFS was seen without a corresponding survival benefit [27].

A large retrospective study of 1933 Korean patients with T-cell lymphomas concluded that addition of etoposide had no progression-free or overall survival benefit, even in younger patients with good performance status. About 17% of the study population consisted of ALCL patients, but there was no differentiation between the ALK-positive and negative subtypes [28].

In summary, the benefit of etoposide comes through predominantly in the ALK-positive ALCL group. For the rest of T-cell lymphomas, etoposide is likely, and active agent and addition of this drug in younger patients remain an option, as long as toxicity can be minimized.

4.2 Role of upfront autologous transplant as consolidation

The PARMA study established the role of high-dose chemotherapy and autologous peripheral stem cell transplant (HDC and APSCT) in relapsed refractory B-cell lymphomas. Given the poor outcomes of T-cell lymphomas, this option was explored in T-cell lymphomas.

One of the earliest prospective studies addressing the role of upfront APSCT in T-cell lymphoma was reported by Corradini et al. [29]. This Italian study reported long-term outcomes of two prospective phase 2 studies of patients with T-cell lymphoma treated with upfront HDC and APSCT. Sixty-two patients with stage 2 to 4 T-cell lymphoma underwent two different conditioning regimens. Thirty percent of these patients had ALK-positive ALCL. Seventy-four percent of the patients underwent HDC and APSCT. Twelve-year overall survival and event-free survival with APSCT were 37 and 25%. ALK-positive ALCL patients had a significantly better survival than their other T-cell lymphoma counterparts. Achieving complete remission (CR) before APSCT was a strong predictor of improved survival in this study. Patients who achieved a CR before transplant had a 12-year DFS of 60% [29].

In another prospective single-arm study, 83 patients with PTCL, AITL, and ALK-negative ALCL as the predominant histologies were treated with 4–6 cycles of CHOP followed by HDC and APSCT. The 3-year OS and PFS were 48 and 36%, respectively. Eighty percent of patients relapsed within 24 months from APSCT [30].

The Nordic lymphoma group conducted a phase 2 prospective trial of 160 patients with T-cell lymphoma, to determine the outcomes of dose-dense chemotherapy followed by HDC and APSCT. Patients were treated with three cycles of CHOPE (cyclophosphamide, doxorubicin, vincristine, prednisolone, and etoposide) every 14 days. In patients older than 60, etoposide was omitted—hence patients received dose-dense CHOP. Those who had partial or complete responses (PR or CR) went on to receive three more cycles of the same chemotherapy regimen followed by HDC and APSCT. Of note, ALK-positive ALCL patients were excluded. PTCL NOS patients were 39% of the cohort, followed by AITL and ALK-negative ALCL, each consisting of 19%. About 70% of patients underwent HDC and APSCT. The 5-year OS and PFS were 51 and 44%, respectively. The ALK-negative ALCL group had the highest 5-year OS of 70%. Toxicities of the dose-dense regimen were however not insignificant. Grades 3 and 4 hematological and non-hematological toxicity rates were 86 and 45%, respectively, with a treatment-related mortality of 4% [31].

While these studies seem to suggest a better outcome with upfront HDC and APSCT, compared to historical controls, the lack of a randomized comparison between upfront HDC and APSCT and conventional chemotherapy alone makes it difficult to establish this as standard of care. Given the absence of randomized trials, HDC and APSCT in first clinical remission (CR1) has been incorporated into guidelines. However, recent data is emerging to suggest that patients in CR1 may actually not benefit from HDC and APSCT.

A retrospective review of 105 patients who received CHOP-based chemotherapy as first-line was done. About 52.1% of the study population were in CR1. About half of these patients underwent HDC and APSCT, whereas the other half were on surveillance. At 22 months, the median PFS of the surveillance group compared to the group that underwent transplant was 15.8 months vs. 12.8 months, but this was not statistically significant. The authors hence concluded that patients who are in CR1 following induction chemotherapy may not benefit from APSCT [32].

Our group did a retrospective analysis of 175 patients from Singapore, South Korea, and China. PTCL NOS patients formed 42% of the cohort. AITL and ALK-negative ALCL formed 33% and 22% of the cohort, respectively. About 92% of patients received anthracycline-based induction chemotherapy. However, only 18% of the cohort underwent upfront HDC and APSCT. Median PFS was 5.5 years for the entire population but OS was not reached. On multivariate analysis, age and advanced stage of disease were identified as poor prognostic factors. The use of anthracycline-based regimens as well as HDC and APSCT did not feature as significant factors affecting survival or progression-free survival outcomes, even in younger patients [33].

These results were echoed in a multicenter retrospective study done in Europe. AITL was the most common subtype in this dataset (46%), compared to PTCL NOS (29%) and ALK-positive ALCL (25%). In order to eliminate selection bias in the retrospective analysis, multivariate proportional hazard model and propensity score matching model were both applied. Two-hundred sixty-nine patients were analyzed among whom half the patients had undergone HDC and APSCT at CR1 and the other half was under surveillance. Five-year PFS and OS were 45% and 60%, respectively, for the overall population. Consolidation APSCT at CR1 did not improve survival outcomes in this population. Once again, remission status (CR or PR) at the end of induction featured as a significant prognostic factor [34].

In summary, achieving a CR at the end of induction therapy is a crucial prognostic factor in determining outcomes in TCL. The role of upfront autologous transplant, especially in patients who have achieved CR1, remains to be defined.

4.3 Role of allogenic transplant in CR1

Two prospective studies attempted to explore the role of allogenic transplant in first remission [35, 36]. In both the studies, about 39% of patients did not undergo transplant, predominantly due to early progression. In the Italian study, only a quarter of the patients who underwent transplant remained in CR at 44 months. Hence, allogenic transplant as consolidation therapy is not recommended.

4.4 Relapsed or refractory disease

In the relapsed setting, autologous or allogenic transplant remains as options following salvage chemotherapy to attain a response. The Center for International Blood and Marrow Transplant Research reported 3-year PFS and OS rates of 41 and 53%, respectively, for patients undergoing autologous transplant at first relapse. The rationale for allogenic transplant in lymphoma has been to harness the graft versus lymphoma effect. Three-year OS for myeloablative versus a non-myeloablative regimen was 31 and 50%, respectively. Once again, having a chemosensitive disease and having two lines of treatment or fewer were important prognostic factors for survival [37, 38].

4.5 Novel agents

4.5.1 Brentuximab vedotin

Brentuximab vedotin is an antibody-drug conjugate (ADC) composed of a chimeric monoclonal antibody linked to an anti-tubulin agent, monomethyl auristatin E (MMAE). The monoclonal antibody targets CD30-expressing cells, and MMAE is released intracellularly to bind to tubulin. The binding of MMAE to tubulin disrupts the microtubule network, causing cell cycle arrest and apoptosis. Brentuximab vedotin is cell cycle phase-specific (G2/M phase). CD30 is uniformly expressed in anaplastic large cell lymphomas. In addition to that, about 43% of PTCL (excluding ALL) has been estimated to have CD30 expression [39].

A phase 2 study demonstrated a response rate of 41% when brentuximab was administered to CD30-positive T-cell lymphomas, at 1.8 mg/kg every 3 weeks. This study excluded ALCL patients. This was a considerable response given that 63% of patients were refractory to the most recent therapy prior to brentuximab. Interestingly, the degree of CD30 expression did not correlate with the responses [40].

A retrospective French study analyzed the effectiveness of brentuximab in 56 patients. Twenty-four patients had ALCL. Cutaneous lymphomas (72%) and

ALCLs (62%) had better overall response rates than non-ALCL PTCLs (21%). Contrary to the study by Horwitz et al., this study reported a statistically significant improvement in PFS with stronger (>75%) expression of CD30 [41].

A prior study in JCO reported exceptional response rates of 86% with the use of brentuximab in relapsed refractory ALCL. The CR rates were 57% and median duration of response was 12.6 months. These excellent responses were demonstrated despite 62% of patients having primary refractory disease [42].

The ALCANZA trial was a phase 3 trial that compared brentuximab against physician choice treatment for patients with cutaneous T-cell lymphomas who have seen prior treatment. This study demonstrated that patients who had brentuximab had better objective global response rates (56.3%) than those who had physician choice treatment (12.5%). The endpoint of objective global response comprised of response in the skin, node, viscera, and blood, lasting for a minimum of 4 months. The median progression-free survival was 16.7 months vs. 3.5 months HR 0.27 ($p < 0.0001$). These results are certainly promising, especially given that this group of diseases has limited efficacious systemic treatment [43, 44].

The efficacy of brentuximab in the relapsed refractory settings has prompted the evaluation of this drug in the first-line setting. A phase 1 study explored the safety and efficacy of combining brentuximab with cyclophosphamide, doxorubicin, and prednisolone (BV CHP) in 26 treatment naïve PTCL patients. Patients received six cycles of BV CHP followed by BV maintenance for up to 10 cycles. Seventy-three percent of the study population consisted of ALCL. One hundred percent response rate with 50% continuing to remain in CR at 5 years was reported. The predominant toxicity was peripheral neuropathy which resolved in the majority. While the results are exciting, it is possible that the results were driven primarily by the ALCL population. A larger randomized study stratified by tumor subtypes will be important before this is adopted as the new standard of care [44].

Regardless, the promising efficacy of brentuximab, at least in the post first-line setting cannot be disregarded. This is generally a well-tolerated drug with predominant toxicities being peripheral neuropathy, myelosuppression, fatigue, and nausea.

4.5.2 Pralatrexate

Pralatrexate is a novel antifolate drug which inhibits dihydrofolate reductase enzyme, thereby inhibiting the conversion of dihydrofolate to tetrahydrofolate. Blocking this essential step in DNA and RNA synthesis results in cell cycle arrest. In addition, its high affinities for reduced folate carrier and folylpolyglutamate synthase are distinctive features that account for its superior activity compared to other drugs in the same class [45]. The early phase II-I-II study showed an overall response rate of 54% in TCL, compared to only 5% in B-cell lymphomas [46]. A weekly dose of 30 mg/m^2 for 6 out of 7 weeks had a better toxicity profile than a dose of 135 mg/m^2 given every other week. The PROPEL study which recruited 115 patients with TCL demonstrated an overall response rate of 29%. Eleven percent achieved CR. Of note, 5 out of 26 patients who were refractory to prior lines of therapy responded to this drug [47]. However, common toxicities of this drug include mucositis, fatigue, myelosuppression, and abnormal liver function tests.

4.5.3 Romidepsin

Romidepsin is predominantly a class 1 histone deacetylase inhibitor (HDAC). Through complex interactions, which remain to be fully understood, this drug disrupts chromatin structure and activates transcription factors. As a result, it mediates cell cycle arrest and cell death and increases transcription of tumor suppressor genes. In a pivotal phase 2 study, romidepsin was administered at 14 mg/m^2 on days 1 and 8 and 15 in a 28 days cycle, to patients with relapsed or refractory T-cell lymphoma. PTCL and AITL were the most common subtypes in the study. A 25% response rate was reported, with 15% achieving CR. Responses were also durable with median duration of response being 17 months [48]. Another phase 2 study by the NCI group reported 38% response rates with duration of response being 8.9 months [49]. The main toxicities in both these studies were cytopenias, infections, fatigue, and nausea.

4.5.4 Belinostat

Belinostat is a pan-HDAC inhibitor which inhibits classes I, II, and IV HDAC. It facilitates apoptosis and cell cycle arrest in abnormal, transformed cells through complex interactions with cell cycle mechanisms. Based on a phase 2 trial which demonstrated 25% response rates in PTCL, the BELIEF (Belinostat in Patients With Relapsed or Refractory Peripheral T-Cell Lymphoma) trial was conducted. This was a single-arm study where belinostat was administered as an intravenous infusion at a dose of 1000 mg/m^2 on days 1–5 Q21 days, to patients with relapsed or refractory T-cell lymphomas. The study reported a modest objective response rate of 26% with duration of response of 8.3 months. Of note, AITL patients had a higher response rate of 46% than 23% in PTCL patients. The main toxicities were fever, hematological toxicities, nausea, and fatigue [50].

5. Conclusion

T-cell lymphoma has evolved from being one disease to a mixed bag of multiple diseases, each of which is being understood at greater depths now, with the advent of technology and molecular biology. With a better understanding of the disease biologies, the therapeutic armamentarium needs to be developed further in order to improve outcomes from these diseases.

Author details

Nagavalli Somasundaram[1] and Soon Thye Lim[1,2]*

1 National Cancer Center Singapore, Singapore

2 Duke-NUS Medical School, Singapore

*Address all correspondence to: lim.soon.thye@singhealth.com.sg

References

[1] Campo E, Swerdlow SH, Harris NL, Pileri S, Stein H, Jaffe ES. The 2008 WHO classification of lymphoid neoplasms and beyond: Evolving concepts and practical applications. Blood. 2011;**117**(19):5019-5032

[2] Swerdlow SH, Campo E, Pileri SA, Harris NL, Stein H, Siebert R, et al. The 2016 revision of the World Health Organization classification of lymphoid neoplasms. Blood. 2016;**127**(20):2375-2390

[3] Matutes E. The 2017 WHO update on mature T- and natural killer (NK) cell neoplasms. International Journal of Laboratory Hematology. 2018;**40** (Suppl 1):97-103

[4] Tang T, Tay K, Quek R, Tao M, Tan SY, Tan L, et al. Peripheral T-cell lymphoma: Review and updates of current management strategies. Advances in Hematology. 2010;**2010**:624040

[5] Vose J, Armitage J, Weisenburger D. International peripheral T-cell and natural killer/T-cell lymphoma study: Pathology findings and clinical outcomes. Journal of Clinical Oncology. 2008;**26**(25):4124-4130

[6] Au WY, Ma SY, Chim CS, Choy C, Loong F, Lie AK, et al. Clinicopathologic features and treatment outcome of mature T-cell and natural killer-cell lymphomas diagnosed according to the World Health Organization classification scheme: A single center experience of 10 years. Annals of Oncology. 2005;**16**(2):206-214

[7] Lim ST, Hee SW, Quek R, Lim LC, Yap SP, Loong EL, et al. Comparative analysis of extra-nodal NK/T-cell lymphoma and peripheral T-cell lymphoma: Significant differences in clinical characteristics and prognosis. European Journal of Haematology. 2008;**80**(1):55-60

[8] Weisenburger DD, Savage KJ, Harris NL, Gascoyne RD, Jaffe ES, MacLennan KA, et al. Peripheral T-cell lymphoma, not otherwise specified: A report of 340 cases from the International Peripheral T-cell Lymphoma Project. Blood. 2011;**117**(12):3402-3408

[9] Lunning MA, Vose JM. Angioimmunoblastic T-cell lymphoma: The many-faced lymphoma. Blood. 2017;**129**(9):1095-1102

[10] Federico M, Rudiger T, Bellei M, Nathwani BN, Luminari S, Coiffier B, et al. Clinicopathologic characteristics of angioimmunoblastic T-cell lymphoma: Analysis of the international peripheral T-cell lymphoma project. Journal of Clinical Oncology. 2013;**31**(2):240-246

[11] Liu HL, Hoppe RT, Kohler S, Harvell JD, Reddy S, Kim YH. CD30+ cutaneous lymphoproliferative disorders: The Stanford experience in lymphomatoid papulosis and primary cutaneous anaplastic large cell lymphoma. Journal of the American Academy of Dermatology. 2003;**49**(6):1049-1058

[12] Marks DI, Rowntree C. Management of adults with T-cell lymphoblastic leukemia. Blood. 2017;**129**(9):1134-1142

[13] Wilcox RA. Cutaneous T-cell lymphoma: 2017 update on diagnosis, risk-stratification, and management. American Journal of Hematology. 2017;**92**(10):1085-1102

[14] Siegel RS, Pandolfino T, Guitart J, Rosen S, Kuzel TM. Primary cutaneous T-cell lymphoma: Review and current concepts. Journal of Clinical Oncology. 2000;**18**(15):2908-2925

[15] Au WY, Pang A, Choy C, Chim CS, Kwong YL. Quantification of circulating

Epstein-Barr virus (EBV) DNA in the diagnosis and monitoring of natural killer cell and EBV-positive lymphomas in immunocompetent patients. Blood. 2004;**104**(1):243-249

[16] Feeney J, Horwitz S, Gonen M, Schoder H. Characterization of T-cell lymphomas by FDG PET/CT. American Journal of Roentgenology. 2010;**195**(2):333-340

[17] Zhou X, Lu K, Geng L, Li X, Jiang Y, Wang X. Utility of PET/CT in the diagnosis and staging of extranodal natural killer/T-cell lymphoma: A systematic review and meta-analysis. Medicine. 2014;**93**(28):e258

[18] Briski R, Feldman AL, Bailey NG, Lim MS, Ristow K, Habermann TM, et al. The role of front-line anthracycline-containing chemotherapy regimens in peripheral T-cell lymphomas. Blood Cancer Journal. 2014;**4**:e214

[19] Yamaguchi M, Kita K, Miwa H, Nishii K, Oka K, Ohno T, et al. Frequent expression of P-glycoprotein/MDR1 by nasal T-cell lymphoma cells. Cancer. 1995;**76**(11):2351-2356

[20] Ando M, Sugimoto K, Kitoh T, Sasaki M, Mukai K, Ando J, et al. Selective apoptosis of natural killer-cell tumours by L-asparaginase. British Journal of Haematology. 2005;**130**(6):860-868

[21] Escalon MP, Liu NS, Yang Y, Hess M, Walker PL, Smith TL, et al. Prognostic factors and treatment of patients with T-cell non-Hodgkin lymphoma: The M. D. Anderson Cancer Center experience. Cancer. 2005;**103**(10):2091-2098

[22] Simon A, Peoch M, Casassus P, Deconinck E, Colombat P, Desablens B, et al. Upfront VIP-reinforced-ABVD (VIP-rABVD) is not superior to CHOP/21 in newly diagnosed peripheral T cell lymphoma. Results of the randomized phase III trial GOELAMS-LTP95. British Journal of Haematology. 2010;**151**(2):159-166

[23] Gleeson M, Peckitt C, To YM, Edwards L, Oates J, Wotherspoon A, et al. CHOP versus GEM-P in previously untreated patients with peripheral T-cell lymphoma (CHEMO-T): A phase 2, multicentre, randomised, open-label trial. The Lancet Haematology. 2018;**5**(5):e190-e200

[24] Pfreundschuh M, Trumper L, Kloess M, Schmits R, Feller AC, Rudolph C, et al. Two-weekly or 3-weekly CHOP chemotherapy with or without etoposide for the treatment of young patients with good-prognosis (normal LDH) aggressive lymphomas: Results of the NHL-B1 trial of the DSHNHL. Blood. 2004;**104**(3):626-633

[25] Pfreundschuh M, Trumper L, Kloess M, Schmits R, Feller AC, Rube C, et al. Two-weekly or 3-weekly CHOP chemotherapy with or without etoposide for the treatment of elderly patients with aggressive lymphomas: Results of the NHL-B2 trial of the DSHNHL. Blood. 2004;**104**(3):634-641

[26] Schmitz N, Trumper L, Ziepert M, Nickelsen M, Ho AD, Metzner B, et al. Treatment and prognosis of mature T-cell and NK-cell lymphoma: An analysis of patients with T-cell lymphoma treated in studies of the German High-Grade Non-Hodgkin Lymphoma Study Group. Blood. 2010;**116**(18):3418-3425

[27] Ellin F, Landstrom J, Jerkeman M, Relander T. Real-world data on prognostic factors and treatment in peripheral T-cell lymphomas: A study from the Swedish Lymphoma Registry. Blood. 2014;**124**(10):1570-1577

[28] Kim YA, Byun JM, Park K, Bae GH, Lee D, Kim DS, et al. Redefining the role of etoposide in first-line treatment

of peripheral T-cell lymphoma. Blood Advances. 2017;**1**(24):2138-2146

[29] Corradini P, Tarella C, Zallio F, Dodero A, Zanni M, Valagussa P, et al. Long-term follow-up of patients with peripheral T-cell lymphomas treated up-front with high-dose chemotherapy followed by autologous stem cell transplantation. Leukemia. 2006;**20**(9):1533-1538

[30] Reimer P, Rudiger T, Geissinger E, Weissinger F, Nerl C, Schmitz N, et al. Autologous stem-cell transplantation as first-line therapy in peripheral T-cell lymphomas: Results of a prospective multicenter study. Journal of Clinical Oncology. 2009;**27**(1):106-113

[31] d'Amore F, Relander T, Lauritzsen GF, Jantunen E, Hagberg H, Anderson H, et al. Up-front autologous stem-cell transplantation in peripheral T-cell lymphoma: NLG-T-01. Journal of Clinical Oncology. 2012;**30**(25):3093-3099

[32] Yam C, Landsburg DJ, Lin X, Mato A, Svoboda J, Loren A, et al. Autologous stem cell transplantation in first complete remission may not extend progression free survival in patients with ALK-negative peripheral T cell lymphoma. Blood. 2015;**126**(23):3183

[33] Tang T, Khoo LP, Lim C, Ham JS, Kim SJ, Hong H, et al. Outcomes of patients with peripheral T-cell lymphoma in first complete remission: Data from three tertiary Asian cancer centers. Blood Cancer Journal. 2017;**7**(12):653

[34] Fossard G, Broussais F, Coelho I, Bailly S, Nicolas-Virelizier E, Toussaint E, et al. Role of up-front autologous stem-cell transplantation in peripheral T-cell lymphoma for patients in response after induction: An analysis of patients from LYSA centers. Annals of Oncology. 2018;**29**(3):715-723

[35] Corradini P, Vitolo U, Rambaldi A, Miceli R, Patriarca F, Gallamini A, et al. Intensified chemo-immunotherapy with or without stem cell transplantation in newly diagnosed patients with peripheral T-cell lymphoma. Leukemia. 2014;**28**(9):1885-1891

[36] Schmitz N, Nickelsen M, Altmann B, Ziepert M, Bouabdallah K, Gisselbrecht C, et al. Allogeneic or autologous transplantation as first-line therapy for younger patients with peripheral T-cell lymphoma: Results of the interim analysis of the AATT trial. Journal of Clinical Oncology. 2015;**33**(15_suppl):8507

[37] Smith SM, Burns LJ, Besien K, LeRademacher J, He W, Fenske TS, et al. Hematopoietic cell transplantation for systemic mature T-cell non-Hodgkin lymphoma. Journal of Clinical Oncology. 2013;**31**(25):3100-3109

[38] Schmitz N, Lenz G, Stelljes M. Allogeneic hematopoietic stem cell transplantation for T-cell lymphomas. Blood. 2018;**132**(3):245-253

[39] Sabattini E, Pizzi M, Tabanelli V, Baldin P, Sacchetti CS, Agostinelli C, et al. CD30 expression in peripheral T-cell lymphomas. Haematologica. 2013;**98**(8):e81-e82

[40] Horwitz SM, Advani RH, Bartlett NL, Jacobsen ED, Sharman JP, O'Connor OA, et al. Objective responses in relapsed T-cell lymphomas with single-agent brentuximab vedotin. Blood. 2014;**123**(20):3095-3100

[41] Lamarque M, Bossard C, Contejean A, Brice P, Parrens M, Le Gouill S, et al. Brentuximab vedotin in refractory or relapsed peripheral T-cell lymphomas: The French named patient program experience in 56 patients. Haematologica. 2016;**101**(3):e103-e106

[42] Pro B, Advani R, Brice P, Bartlett NL, Rosenblatt JD, Illidge T, et al. Brentuximab

vedotin (SGN-35) in patients with relapsed or refractory systemic anaplastic large-cell lymphoma: Results of a phase II study. Journal of Clinical Oncology. 2012;**30**(18):2190-2196

[43] Prince HM, Kim YH, Horwitz SM, Dummer R, Scarisbrick J, Quaglino P, et al. Brentuximab vedotin or physician's choice in CD30-positive cutaneous T-cell lymphoma (ALCANZA): An international, open-label, randomised, phase 3, multicentre trial. Lancet (London, England). 2017;**390**(10094):555-566

[44] Prince HM, Gautam A, Kim YH. Brentuximab vedotin: Targeting CD30 as standard in CTCL. Oncotarget. 2018;**9**(15):11887-11888

[45] Marchi E, Mangone M, Zullo K, O'Connor OA. Pralatrexate pharmacology and clinical development. Clinical Cancer Research. 2013;**19**(24):6657-6661

[46] O'Connor OA, Horwitz S, Hamlin P, Portlock C, Moskowitz CH, Sarasohn D, et al. Phase II-I-II study of two different doses and schedules of pralatrexate, a high-affinity substrate for the reduced folate carrier, in patients with relapsed or refractory lymphoma reveals marked activity in T-cell malignancies. Journal of Clinical Oncology. 2009;**27**(26):4357-4364

[47] O'Connor OA, Pro B, Pinter-Brown L, Bartlett N, Popplewell L, Coiffier B, et al. Pralatrexate in patients with relapsed or refractory peripheral T-cell lymphoma: Results from the pivotal PROPEL study. Journal of Clinical Oncology. 2011;**29**(9):1182-1189

[48] Coiffier B, Pro B, Prince HM, Foss F, Sokol L, Greenwood M, et al. Results from a pivotal, open-label, phase II study of romidepsin in relapsed or refractory peripheral T-cell lymphoma after prior systemic therapy. Journal of Clinical Oncology. 2012;**30**(6):631-636

[49] Piekarz RL, Frye R, Prince HM, Kirschbaum MH, Zain J, Allen SL, et al. Phase 2 trial of romidepsin in patients with peripheral T-cell lymphoma. Blood. 2011;**117**(22):5827-5834

[50] Sawas A, Radeski D, O'Connor OA. Belinostat in patients with refractory or relapsed peripheral T-cell lymphoma: A perspective review. Therapeutic Advances in Hematology. 2015;**6**(4):202-208

Chapter 3

Anaplastic Large Cell Lymphoma

Suzanne D. Turner

Abstract

Anaplastic large cell lymphoma (ALCL) describes a distinct group of T cell lymphomas characterised by cell surface expression of CD30. At least three entities of ALCL exist, with similar cellular morphology but varying clinical courses and pathology: systemic ALCL, anaplastic lymphoma kinase (ALK)-positive, systemic ALCL ALK− and primary cutaneous ALCL. A fourth provisional entity associated with breast implants has been proposed, named breast implant-associated (BIA)-ALCL. ALCL have varying clinical outcomes, affect both children and adults, and range from being well-characterised at the genetic level to relatively unknown, predominantly due to the relative rarity of this group of malignancies. Current therapeutic approaches include standard chemotherapeutic agents as well as novel drugs including monoclonal antibodies and kinase inhibitors.

Keywords: anaplastic large cell lymphoma, anaplastic lymphoma kinase, tyrosine kinase inhibitors, peripheral T cell lymphoma, BIA-ALCL

1. Introduction

Anaplastic large cell lymphoma (ALCL) was first described in 1985 as a CD30-positive (or ki-1+) histiocytic lymphoma, later re-classified as a distinct clinical entity, ALCL [1]. The presence of a chromosomal translocation in this malignancy was described independently by several authors in 1989–1990 [2–5]. This was further refined in 1994 on cloning of the t(2;5)(p23;q35) translocation breakpoint product, identified as a fusion protein of Nucleophosmin 1 (NPM) and anaplastic lymphoma kinase (ALK), the latter a previously uncharacterized protein named after the disease from which it was cloned [6]. Sometime later in 2008, systemic (s) ALCL was divided into two provisional entities: ALCL, ALK+ and ALCL, ALK− which were confirmed as distinct entities in the revised 4th edition of the WHO classification of tumours of haemopoietic and lymphoid tissues [7]. The revised 4th edition also includes a new provisional entity of ALCL associated with breast implants, breast implant-associated (BIA)-ALCL which may consist of at least two clinically distinguishable forms, if not a spectrum of disease, ranging from sub-capsular seroma fluid to aggressive, infiltrating masses with good and poor prognoses respectively [8, 9]. As well as systemic forms of the disease, there exists a cutaneous type belonging to the class of primary cutaneous CD30-positive T cell lymphoproliferative disorders—primary cutaneous (pc) ALCL [7]. In this chapter, the clinical and pathological presentations of each of these disease entities will be presented and discussed as will the biology underlying these malignancies.

2. Systemic ALCL

2.1 Clinical course

The large majority of ALCL, ALK+ are diagnosed in a younger patient population with a median age of 10.2–11 and have a relatively good prognosis (>80% overall survival; OS) [10–15]. In contrast ALCL, ALK– more often affects an older demographic (40–65 years of age) and has a poor prognosis (<50% OS) [16–19]. Whether these different clinical outcomes are age-related or due to inherent properties of the malignancies remains to be determined although in support of the latter, ALK– ALCL carrying DUSP22 rearrangements have been reported to have a superior 5-year OS of 90% (compared to 17% for TP63 rearranged cases and 42% for ALK–/DUSP22–/TP63– cases) although if patients are stratified according to age rather than ALK status, the outcome in response to treatment is the same [17, 19, 20]. The relatively high survival rates of patients diagnosed with ALCL, ALK+ may also be attributable to the host immune response whereby cytotoxic T lymphocytes, helper T cells and B cells responding to ALK have been detected in patients [21, 22]. Patients with ALCL, ALK+ mount an immune response to the ALK protein in the form of a humoral antibody response [23]. In fact, the titre of ALK autoantibodies in a patient's serum can be predictive of outcome with an inverse correlation between ALK antibodies and relapse [24]. This prognostic factor can be extended further when combined with the presence or absence of minimal disseminated disease (MDD), with children having low ALK autoantibody titres combined with presence of MDD being of high risk, with the converse indicative of low risk [25].

2.2 Histopathological presentation and immunophenotype

ALCL spans a broad morphological spectrum with sub-types including common (65%), small cell and lymphohistiocytic variants (32% combined) with the latter constituting a poor prognostic variable [26–28]. The unifying feature of ALCL is the presence of CD30 expression on the surface of the tumour cells, particularly the larger ones. CD30 is a marker of activated immune cells but does not distinguish between a T or B cell origin when applied in isolation. Hence, for a diagnosis of a T cell lymphoma, a cell surface protein, or combination of proteins unique to T cells must be detected. In this regard, many ALCL express CD4, CD2 and/or CD5 but often lack CD3. The positive expression of CD4 in the absence of CD8 combined with the presence of cytotoxic proteins such as TIA-1, Granzyme B and/or perforin is at odds with the presumed cytotoxic T cell origin of ALCL [7, 29]. However, in some cases, no T cell specific proteins are detectable and these are categorised as being 'null cell', although the majority demonstrate molecular rearrangements of the T cell receptor (TCR) [30].

2.3 Underlying genetic alterations

2.3.1 ALCL, ALK+

ALCL is, in general, a genetically stable cancer with few common defining genetic alterations besides translocations involving ALK [31, 32]. In this regard, the t(2;5)(p23;q35) generating NPM-ALK at the breakpoint is the most common event with many variants having been published over the years (**Table 1**) [33]. The common expression of NPM-ALK, and its nuclear and cytoplasmic location as opposed to cytoplasmic-alone position as seen with many of the other variants, may account for its predominance in ALCL, ALK+; nuclear location may provide a competitive advantage over cytoplasmic alone. Alternatively, the *NPM1* gene on chromosome 5 may be

Chromosomal alteration	Fusion protein	Cellular location	References
t(2;5)(p23;q35)	NPM-ALK	Nucleus and cytoplasm	[2–6]
t(2;3)(p23;q12.2)	TFG-ALK (short, long and extra-long isoforms)	Cytoplasm	[134, 135]
t(1;2)(q25;p23)	TPM3-ALK	Cytoplasm	[136]
Inv(2)(p23;q35)	ATIC-ALK	Cytoplasm	[137, 138]
t(X;2)(q11–12;p23)	MSN-ALK	Membrane	[139]
t(2;17)(p23;q23)	CLTC-ALK	Cytoplasm (granular)	[140, 141]
t(2;22)(p23;q11.2)	MYH9-ALK	Cytoplasm	[142]
t(2;19)(p23;q13.1)	TPM4-ALK	Cytoplasm	[143]
t(2;17)(p23;q25)	RNF213/ALO17-ALK	Cytoplasm	[144]

Table 1.
Overview of ALK fusion partners identified in ALCL, ALK+.

more prone to breakage and fusion with new partners due to its active transcription at the same time as *ALK*, although there is no evidence to suggest this is the case. What is clear, is that all reported ALK fusion proteins generate a hyperactive tyrosine kinase that is ligand-independent, driving cellular proliferation and survival [33]. Taking the example of NPM-ALK, this fusion protein retains the oligomerisation domains of NPM1 and the entire intracellular portion of ALK encoding the kinase domain, resulting in dimerization, auto-phosphorylation and subsequent hyperactivity initiating a whole plethora of signal transduction pathways (**Figure 1**) [6, 34].

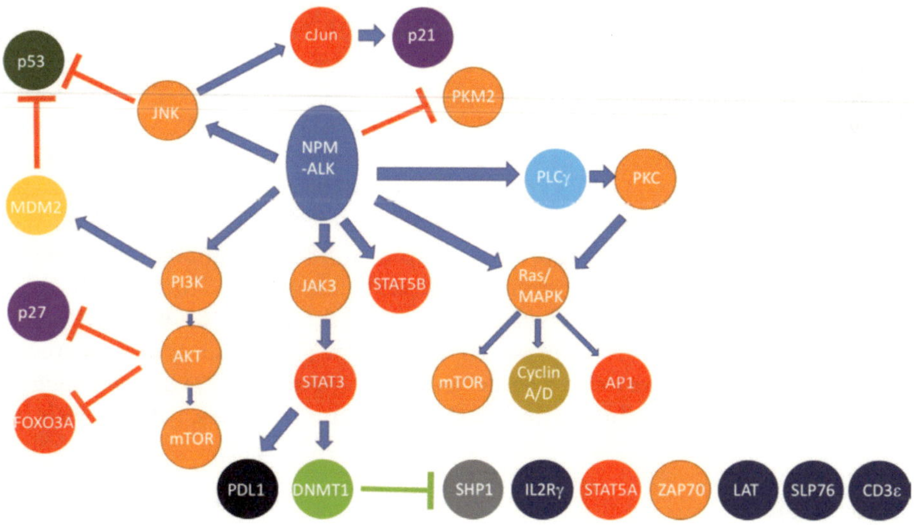

Figure 1.
NPM-ALK activates a plethora of signalling pathways conferring many of the cancer hallmarks on tumour cells. NPM-ALK autophosphorylates tyrosine residues providing docking sites for SH2 domain-containing proteins and the development of a signalosome consisting of at least 46 proteins [35]. Key pathways involved in cell survival and proliferation include the PI 3-Kinase/Akt, Ras/MAP Kinase and JAK/STAT pathways as well as PLCγ [36–41]. While activation of JNK and PI 3-Kinase by NPM-ALK can drive cell proliferation, they also inactivate p53 by ubiquitin-mediated degradation [42]. NPM-ALK also activates immunomodulatory pathways including up-regulation of PDL1 mediated by STAT3, as well as silencing some proteins by epigenetic means (green arrow, **Figure 1***), including those associated with signalling downstream of a functional TCR [43–47]. In addition, NPM-ALK directs metabolic activity of the cells shifting to aerobic glycolysis with increased lactate and biomass production promoting cell survival [48].*

While ALK translocations are diagnostic of ALCL, ALK+ and are central to disease pathogenesis, the role of other contributing mutations is largely unknown as few consistent genetic abnormalities besides those generating ALK translocations have been reported. This may, in part, be due to the plethora a cancer hallmarks that can be driven by NPM-ALK alone (**Figure 1**). However, array comparative genomic hybridization (aCGH) studies have highlighted some commonalities [31, 32]. For example, gains of chromosomes 7, 6q, 17p, 17q24-qter and losses of chromosomes 4q13-q21, 11q14 and 13q although the significance of these is unknown [32]. However, a higher number of genomic imbalances as detected by aCGH at a resolution of 1 MB, has been associated with a worse prognosis [31].

The recognition of NPM-ALK as a driving oncogenic event and the paucity of other reported consistent genomic/genetic abnormalities in ALCL, ALK+ has led to studies of the epigenetics of ALCL [31, 49, 50]. Profiling of CpG methylation in ALCL defined a number of genes silenced in these malignancies including the TCR signalling-related proteins Zap70, LAT, CD3ε, SLP76 and the IL2Rγ chain [43, 45–47, 49, 51]. Given that NPM-ALK can substitute for signalling normally induced via an engaged TCR, activation of these proximal TCR signalling proteins may be detrimental to cell survival resulting in their evolutionary down-regulation [38, 52]. Furthermore, a number of miRNA have been implicated in tumorigenesis including miR17-92, miR135b, miR29a and miR16 [53–56].

2.3.2 ALCL, ALK−

By their very definition, ALCL, ALK− lack expression of ALK fusion proteins, but until recently, few studies had found major contributory and consistent mutations. DUSP22 rearrangements leading to loss of expression of DUSP22 have been reported in as many as 30% of cases and activating *JAK1/STAT3* mutations in 20% [19, 57, 58]. In addition, rearrangements leading to *TP63* mutation (8% of cases) and ERBB4 truncation have been demonstrated as have novel, rare rearrangements leading to the generation of NcoR2-ROS1, NFkB2-ROS1 and NFkB2-TYK2 fusion proteins [19, 57, 59, 60]. In addition, similar to ALK+ ALCL, miRNA have been implicated in disease pathogenesis including miR155 as well as others that enable a molecular distinction between ALCL, ALK+ and ALK− as well as peripheral T cell lymphoma, not otherwise specified (PTCL-NOS) [61–64]. Likewise, genomic classifiers of ALCL, ALK− amongst other peripheral T cell lymphomas have been demonstrated using a variety of genomic analysis techniques and includes the differentiating 3-gene signature of *TNFRSF8*, *BATF3* and *TMOD1* [65–68]. SNP arrays have also led to the identification of recurrent losses at 17p13 and/or 6q21 where the *TP53* and *PRDM1* genes are located respectively, in as many as 52% of cases suggestive of a role for the loss of the p53 and BLIMP1 proteins in disease pathogenesis [69].

3. BIA-ALCL

BIA-ALCL is a relatively new addition to the spectrum of ALCL, although the first case was reported in 1997, but did not receive much attention until further cases were identified and published, and the FDA acknowledged an association in 2011 [70, 71]. In March 2015, the French health minister issued a warning following reports of 18 cases in France [72]. A further follow-up report released by the FDA in 2017 described 414 medical device reports and 9 deaths associated with BIA-ALCL [73]. Many case series have been reviewed and reported since, with data from France, Italy,

The Netherlands, UK, Australia and the USA being prevalent [74–80]. Most recently, seven cases have been reported in Latin America [81]. There are approximately 5–10 million women with breast implants worldwide with rates of BIA-ALCL being proportionately rare although difficult to put an exact figure to. Dependent on the study conducted, incidence rates range from 1 to 89 cases per million women with breast implants [82, 83]. This reaches a much higher incidence if one considers women with textured implants alone. Almost all cases reported to date have been associated with a breast implant of a textured surface at some point during the history of the patient; whilst rare cases have been reported in women with smooth implants, the patient had been in receipt of a textured implant at some stage [78, 84]. In addition, both saline and silicone filled implants have been implicated in patients with BIA-ALCL. The tumour cells generally present as a monoclonal expansion of CD30-positive cells, as an effusion within the fibrous capsule surrounding the implant [78].

3.1 Clinical course

BIA-ALCL appears to represent at least two clinical entities if not a spectrum of malignancies; patients present on most occasions with an indolent seroma with rarer incidences of invasive solid masses [77]. Indeed, cases have been reported of tumour growth into the ribs with metastases to distant lymph nodes [85, 86].

3.2 Histopathological presentation and immunophenotype

Like sALCL, BIA-ALCL is characterised by CD30 expression on lymphoid cells, in the latter situation contained within the peri-prosthetic effusion [28, 87]. These cells can be detected by immunohistochemistry, cytology and flow cytometry of seroma fluid or any solid mass [85]. A Th17/Th1 origin has been proposed whereby tumour cells secrete IFNγ, IL6, IL8, IL17 and TGFβ although a Th2 derivation has also been put forward [88–90].

3.3 Underlying genetic alterations

Like ALCL, ALK−, BIA-ALCL has not to date been associated with genomic events leading to activation of ALK. However, in concert with ALCL, ALK−, activating mutations of JAK/STAT proteins have been reported in a very few cases [91, 92]. Given the relative rarity of this disease, larger scale studies are required to elucidate the underlying genetics.

4. Primary cutaneous ALCL

While skin involvement can occur as an extranodal manifestation of sALCL, isolated cutaneous disease can also occur, although this is largely ALK-negative [17]. Primary cutaneous ALCL belongs to the spectrum of CD30 positive lymphoproliferative disorders (LPDs) and like BIA-ALCL is largely indolent in nature. While largely affecting adults who present with isolated, ulcerating nodules, children can also develop pcALCL.

4.1 Clinical course

Like systemic ALCL, ALK−, cutaneous ALCL is also a disease of an older demographic with the majority of patients being over 50 years of age, yet is closer to ALCL, ALK+ in its prognosis, reaching a 5-year OS of over 90% [17]. However, relapse is relatively common in this patient group occurring in as many as 30–40% of patients and some rare cases (12–16%) can progress to systemic disease [93–95]. Spontaneous regression has been reported, although in rare cases with partial regressions being more common [96].

4.2 Histopathological presentation and immunophenotype

Diagnosis can be difficult with other cutaneous T cell lymphomas such as lymphomatoid papulosis (LyP) and transformed mycosis fungoides (MF) providing differential diagnoses [9]. However, like systemic ALCL, CD30 expression is a defining feature of this malignancy as it is for the other CD30-associated LPDs.

4.3 Underlying genetic alterations

Due to its relative rarity, sometimes-difficult diagnosis and indolent course, studies of the underlying genetics are few. However, limited studies have elucidated some of the genetic events that may be driving this disease process some of which are also common to sALCL. For example, as in sALCL, DUSP22-IRF4 rearrangements have been detected in 20–57% of pcALCL and ALK expression is seen in rare cases [19, 97–101]. In addition, aCGH has identified gains of 7q31 and losses of 6q16-21 as well as 13q34, collectively in 45% of examined patient specimens [102]. As well as similarities to ALCL, ALK-negative with regards to DUSP22 translocations, upregulation of miR155 has also been observed in both pcALCL and sALCL, ALK– [61, 103]. The functional and clinical significance of these genetic events is still subject to investigation.

5. Treatment of ALCL

As for most peripheral T cell lymphomas, standard combination chemotherapy has been the mainstay of treatment for many years, specifically in the case of systemic disease [14]. In contrast, the relatively indolent cutaneous and breast implant-associated forms are primarily treated by surgical removal [86]. However, as this spectrum of diseases crosses age boundaries, there are age-specific differences in therapeutic approaches.

5.1 Treatment of children with ALCL

As mentioned before, the large majority of patients diagnosed with ALCL, ALK+ are children and young adults. As such, the therapeutic approach is tuned to this patient population with children receiving a combination of chemotherapeutic agents with survival rates in excess of 90% [10, 13, 14]. The ALCL99 trial, the largest trial ever to be conducted for children diagnosed with ALCL (n = 352) applied a therapeutic regimen consisting of a B cell protocol (based on NHL-BFM-B) with randomisation of vinblastine [13]. The success of this trial has led to most centres adopting the ALCL99 treatment protocol. Additionally, the success of the ALCL99 trial and the plethora of biological data produced suggest that patients might be stratified according to ALK autoantibody titre and the presence of MDD as discussed above. Indeed, vinblastine monotherapy might be more appropriate for low risk patients reducing both acute and chronic side-effects of the combination chemotherapy protocol [104, 105].

5.2 Treatment of adults with ALCL

Adults with ALCL tend to be ALK− and are treated with the standard T cell lymphoma regimen CHOP (cyclophosphamide, doxorubicin, vincristine, prednisone) although CHOEP (CHOP + etoposide) has been demonstrated to be superior in the treatment of adult ALCL, ALK+ patients [106]. In the case of BIA-ALCL, surgical excision with complete capsulectomy is recommended and is often sufficient to induce remission particularly for patients that present with a contained seroma [85, 86]. However, patients with aggressive BIA-ALCL that has metastasised require radiotherapy if not chemotherapy, and anecdotal evidence suggests that upfront use of brentuximab vedotin (BV) may benefit these patients [107]. In the case of pcALCL, localised excision and/or radiotherapy is largely prescribed due to the obvious skin presentation, although cases with multi-focal lesions may require more aggressive treatment involving chemotherapy [108, 109].

5.3 New and novel treatment options for ALCL

In the post-genomic era, targeted agents have become the mainstay of chemotherapy, largely in addition to standard cytotoxic drugs. In the case of ALCL, ALK+, inhibitors of ALK are the obvious choice and many have been developed since the discovery of ALK expression in Non-Small Cell Lung Cancer [14]. The first ALK inhibitor to be developed was Pfizer's PF-2341066, now known as crizotinib, a dual ALK/cMet inhibitor with efficacy in experimental models of ALCL, ALK+ [110]. However, these drugs have been slow to make their way into the clinic for the treatment of ALCL, largely due to its relative rarity and paediatric presentation. A phase I study of crizotinib for children with relapsed/refractory ALK+ malignancies including ALCL, reported seven out of nine patients to achieve a complete response (CR) [111]. A phase II expansion cohort showed overall response rates of 83 and 90% respectively for those children receiving crizotinib at dosages of 165 and 280 mg/m^2 respectively [112]. However, discontinuation of therapy has led to rapid relapse of both children and adults with ALCL, ALK+ questioning the required window of therapy [113].

Naturally, ALK inhibitors only apply to the therapy of ALCL, ALK+. In contrast, the common expression of CD30 on all ALCL sub-types means that targeted agents to this cell surface protein should be broadly applicable [114]. In this vein, BV, an anti-CD30 antibody tethered to the microtubule inhibitor monomethyl auristatin E, has shown promising results in clinical trials, although relapse is again an issue with down-regulation of CD30 expression seen [115–117]. However, results of the Phase 3 ALCANZA trial for pcALCL and MF showed impressive results with an objective response rate of 67% in the BV arm (versus 20% in the standard treatment arm: methotrexate or bexarotene) [118]. However, BV is not without its side-effects with peripheral neuropathy being prominent (affecting 67% of patients in the afore-mentioned trial) [118]. Likewise, results of a Phase 2 trial of relapsed/refractory sALCL showed peripheral neuropathy to be a considerable side-effect in 91% of patients although a 5-year OS of 79% was achieved (69% CR, 80% ORR for ALK+ patients and 52% CR, 81% ORR for ALK−) [119]. A randomised Phase 3 trial to establish the efficacy of BV in combination with cyclophosphamide, doxorubicin and prednisolone, in comparison to these chemotherapeutic agents given with vincristine in place of BV, is ongoing for the frontline treatment of CD30-positive lymphomas including ALCL (ECHELON 2; NCT01777152). Other potential therapeutic targets for the treatment of ALCL include PDGFR, JAK/STAT, PD-1/PDL1 and reactivation of p53 [42, 44, 120, 121].

Indeed, biological studies have identified a number of potential therapeutic targets, which in some cases, and with time, have been matched to available drugs. However, with relatively few patients, coupled with a good prognosis, at least for children with ALK+ systemic disease, it is difficult to formulate trials to test these agents.

A further approach given the immune response to ALK in patients with ALK-positive disease, is a vaccination strategy [122]. This is especially relevant as ALK expression seems to be limited to tissues of neonatal origin suggesting that side-effects will be limited [123].

6. The origins and pathogenesis of ALCL: a common origin with distinct pathogenesis or different origins converging on a shared histopathology?

6.1 Cell of origin

Systemic ALCL presents in the periphery suggestive of a peripheral T cell origin, although as many as 50% of children show mediastinal involvement [29]. In this latter vein, a thymic origin has been proposed whereby gene expression signatures associated with early thymic progenitors (ETP) are detected in ALCL cancer stem cells, in fitting with the detection of transcripts for the t(2;5)(p23;q35) translocation breakpoint product in 2% of cord blood specimens from healthy babies [124, 125]. In addition, studies of epigenetic signatures are in keeping with an ETP origin [49]. As such, it is not inconceivable that ALCL, ALK+ has a thymic, perhaps *in utero* origin in-line with the pathogenesis of paediatric leukaemias [29]. Additionally, this is in keeping with a paediatric presentation and the early-life involution of the thymus. Furthermore, studies of murine models show that events in the periphery once incipient tumour cells emerge from the thymus contribute to disease pathogenesis as discussed below [30].

While ALCL, ALK+ is proposed to emerge from the thymus, a similar origin likely does not apply to ALK-negative disease, including pcALCL, BIA-ALCL and ALCL, ALK−. In these latter cases, circulating peripheral T cells are most probably the cells of origin given the older age of diagnosis and peripheral location, particularly with regards to BIA-ALCL and pcALCL. If this is the case, if the type of T cell that becomes transformed can be identified, this may give clues as to disease pathogenesis. While histopathology indicating an activated CD30-expressing T cell producing cytotoxic proteins, yet also often retaining CD4 expression, has given rise to a presumed cytotoxic T cell origin, recent data challenges this perception [29, 126]. Specifically, analysis of gene expression data suggests a Th17 origin, a T cell that usually responds to large extracellular infectious agents such as bacteria and is often implicated in autoimmune disease [89, 127]. However, given that ALCL often lack expression of TCR-related signalling proteins as well as a functional cell surface TCR, analogies to innate lymphoid cells (ILC), specifically ILC type 3 cells are also apparent [127]. Naturally, the eventual cell phenotype is not necessarily reflective of the cell of origin with environmental events likely contributing to the final observed identity. In this regard, whether in ALCL, ALK+ this is shaped by ALK-mediated activities (or is the consequence of other induced (epi)genetic events) remains to be fully elucidated as it does for other ALCL sub-types. In evidence, it has been shown that NPM-ALK induces expression of cytotoxic proteins suggesting that their presence reflects the activities of this inherent transforming event rather than a property of the cell of origin, at least for ALCL, ALK+ [128]. This would partly explain the 'confused' T cell phenotype with both helper and cytotoxic T cell properties apparent. Indeed, plasticity amongst helper T cell subsets is immense and is dependent on the relative expression levels of key transcription factors such as T-bet, RORγ, GATA-3 and Foxp3 as well as cytokines in the microenvironment [129]. Hence, for a T cell aberrantly expressing a variety of genetic changes, embedded in specific inflammatory microenvironments, the resultant cell surface phenotype may no longer reflect the cell of origin.

Another factor to consider is genetic predisposition or health status of the patients whereby some, with for example, autoimmune disease or allergies and a preponderance of Th17 or Th1/Th2 cells respectively may be more at risk, with the resultant tumour phenotype dependent on this. In evidence, at least for BIA-ALCL Th1, Th2 and Th17 origins have been proposed based on the profile of secreted cytokines and expression of specific transcription factors, although of course none of these factors in isolation are necessarily truly indicative of the cell of origin, and as mentioned before, the contribution of the microenvironment cannot be discounted [88–90].

6.2 An infectious aetiology?

The common expression of CD30 on all entities of ALCL is suggestive of an infectious aetiology whereby activation of the underlying T cells triggers expression of this cell surface protein. However, individual cell surface proteins in isolation are not necessarily indicative of the cell of origin of any given cancer, which combined with the propensity of cancer cells to aberrantly up- or down-regulate expression of proteins according to evolutionary fitness necessitates further evidence to draw conclusive decisions. Yet, in evidence of an infectious aetiology,

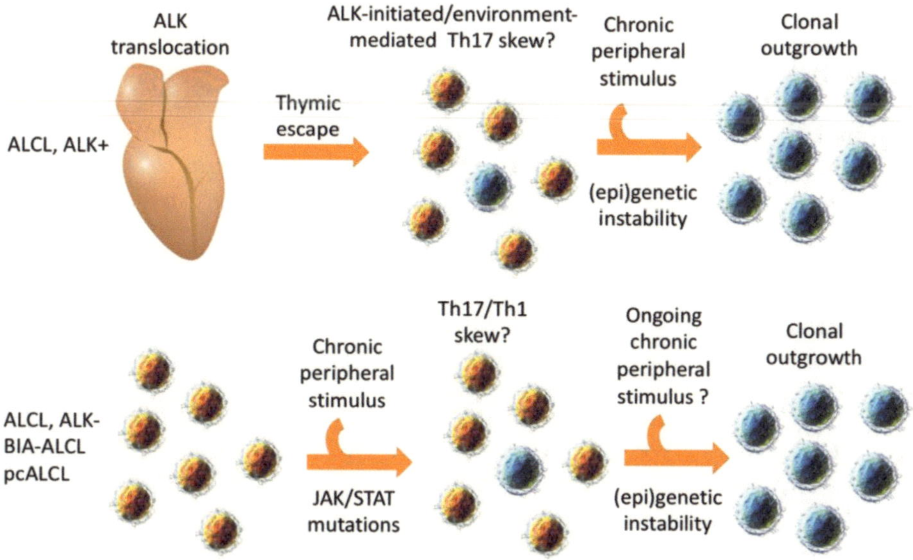

Figure 2.
Proposed mechanisms of tumorigenesis for ALCL. Data suggest that the NPM-ALK generating chromosomal translocation occurs in primitive haemopoietic cells, such as early thymic progenitors, whereby aberrant TCR rearrangements are tolerated [30]. Incipient tumour cells then exit into the periphery where secondary events lead to transformation. Conversely, systemic ALCL, ALK−, pcALCL and BIA-ALCL more likely initiate in circulating peripheral T cells whereby chronic antigenic stimulation mediated by infectious agents, an inflammatory milieu and/or toxic insult leads to the acquisition of malignancy-promoting mutations and cellular transformation.

sALCL have been reported in the context of insect and tick bites, as well as bacterial infections on the surface of breast implants in BIA-ALCL and in association with cutaneous T cell lymphomas whereby TLRs 2, 4 and 7 are expressed by tumour cells [130–132]. Such infectious aetiologies would also produce an inflammatory microenvironment dictated by the infectious agent whereby cytokines, growth factors and many cell types involved in inflammation would be present and may contribute to disease pathogenesis. In this regard, the lymphohistiocytic subtype of sALCL is, as its name suggests, infiltrated with macrophages and many cytokines have been detected at elevated levels in patients diagnosed with ALCL, ALK+ [26, 133] (**Figure 2**).

7. Conclusions

ALCL is a diverse disease entity affecting a range of patients ranging from children to women with breast implants. What is clear, is that all ALCL share some common immunohistopathological features, most prominently CD30 expression, but the clinical courses of these diseases vary considerably from the indolent LPD, pcALCL through to aggressive, poor prognostic malignancies such as sALCL, ALK−. Our understanding of the underlying biology is improving year on year and has had a significant impact on clinical decision making including therapeutic approaches. While for many forms of ALCL, therapy has not altered considerably over the past decade, novel targeted approaches to treatment are entering the clinical arena ranging from monoclonal antibodies to kinase inhibitors. Indeed, we are now in the fortunate position whereby there are a plethora of therapeutic agents, but too few patients to trial them.

Acknowledgements

I would like to acknowledge all authors that have contributed to our understanding of ALCL who could not be cited due to page length restrictions.

Conflict of interest

The author declares no conflicts of interest.

Author details

Suzanne D. Turner
Department of Pathology, University of Cambridge, Cambridge, UK

*Address all correspondence to: sdt36@cam.ac.uk

References

[1] Stein H et al. The expression of the Hodgkin's disease associated antigen Ki-1 in reactive and neoplastic lymphoid tissue: Evidence that Reed-Sternberg cells and histiocytic malignancies are derived from activated lymphoid cells. Blood. 1985;**66**(4):848-858

[2] Kaneko Y et al. A novel translocation, t(2,5)(p23;q35), in childhood phagocytic large T-cell lymphoma mimicking malignant histiocytosis. Blood. 1989;**73**(3):806-813

[3] Le Beau MM et al. The t(2;5)(p23;q35): A recurring chromosomal abnormality in Ki-1-positive anaplastic large cell lymphoma. Leukemia. 1989;**3**(12):866-870

[4] Bitter MA et al. Morphology in Ki-1(CD30)-positive non-Hodgkin's lymphoma is correlated with clinical features and the presence of a unique chromosomal abnormality, t(2;5)(p23;q35). The American Journal of Surgical Pathology. 1990;**14**(4): 305-316

[5] Rimokh R et al. A translocation involving a specific breakpoint (q35) on chromosome 5 is characteristic of anaplastic large cell lymphoma ('Ki-1 lymphoma'). British Journal of Haematology. 1989;**71**(1):31-36

[6] Morris SW et al. Fusion of a kinase gene, ALK, to a nucleolar protein gene, NPM, in non-Hodgkin's lymphoma. Science. 1994;**263**(5151):1281-1284

[7] Swerdlow SH. WHO Classification of Tumours of Haematopoietic and Lymphoid Tissues. Lyon: International Agency for Research on Cancer; 2008. 439 p

[8] Swerdlow SH et al. The 2016 revision of the World Health Organization classification of lymphoid neoplasms. Blood. 2016;**127**(20):2375-2390

[9] Swerdlow SH. World Health Organization, and International Agency for Research on Cancer. In: WHO Classification of Tumours of Haematopoietic and Lymphoid Tissues. Revised 4th ed. World Health Organization Classification of Tumours; 2017. p. 585

[10] Minard-Colin V et al. Non-Hodgkin lymphoma in children and adolescents: Progress through effective collaboration, current knowledge, and challenges ahead. Journal of Clinical Oncology. 2015;**33**(27):2963-2974

[11] Turner SD et al. Anaplastic large cell lymphoma in paediatric and young adult patients. British Journal of Haematology. 2016;**173**(4):560-572

[12] Le Deley MC et al. Prognostic factors in childhood anaplastic large cell lymphoma: Results of a large European intergroup study. Blood. 2008;**111**(3):1560-1566

[13] Le Deley MC et al. Vinblastine in children and adolescents with high-risk anaplastic large-cell lymphoma: Results of the randomized ALCL99-vinblastine trial. Journal of Clinical Oncology. 2010;**28**(25):3987-3993

[14] Prokoph N et al. Treatment options for paediatric anaplastic large cell lymphoma (ALCL): Current standard and beyond. Cancers (Basel). 2018 Mar 30;**10**(4). pii: E99. DOI: 10.3390/cancers10040099

[15] d'Amore ES et al. Anaplastic large cell lymphomas: A study of 75 pediatric patients. Pediatric and Developmental Pathology. 2007;**10**(3):181-191

[16] ten Berge RL et al. ALK-negative anaplastic large-cell lymphoma demonstrates similar poor prognosis to peripheral T-cell lymphoma,

unspecified. Histopathology. 2003;**43**(5):462-469

[17] Savage KJ et al. ALK-anaplastic large-cell lymphoma is clinically and immunophenotypically different from both ALK+ ALCL and peripheral T-cell lymphoma, not otherwise specified: Report from the international peripheral T-cell lymphoma project. Blood. 2008;**111**(12):5496-5504

[18] Gascoyne RD et al. Prognostic significance of anaplastic lymphoma kinase (ALK) protein expression in adults with anaplastic large cell lymphoma. Blood. 1999;**93**(11):3913-3921

[19] Parrilla Castellar ER et al. ALK-negative anaplastic large cell lymphoma is a genetically heterogeneous disease with widely disparate clinical outcomes. Blood. 2014;**124**(9):1473-1480

[20] Sibon D et al. Long-term outcome of adults with systemic anaplastic large-cell lymphoma treated within the Groupe d'Etude des Lymphomes de l'Adulte trials. Journal of Clinical Oncology. 2012;**30**(32):3939-3946

[21] Ait-Tahar K, Barnardo MC, Pulford K. CD4 T-helper responses to the anaplastic lymphoma kinase (ALK) protein in patients with ALK-positive anaplastic large-cell lymphoma. Cancer Research. 2007;**67**(5):1898-1901

[22] Ait-Tahar K et al. B and CTL responses to the ALK protein in patients with ALK-positive ALCL. International Journal of Cancer. 2006;**118**(3): 688-695

[23] Pulford K et al. Immune response to the ALK oncogenic tyrosine kinase in patients with anaplastic large-cell lymphoma. Blood. 2000;**96**(4):1605-1607

[24] Ait-Tahar K et al. Correlation of the autoantibody response to the ALK oncoantigen in pediatric anaplastic lymphoma kinase-positive anaplastic large cell lymphoma with tumor dissemination and relapse risk. Blood. 2010;**115**(16):3314-3319

[25] Mussolin L et al. Kinetics of humoral response to ALK and its relationship with minimal residual disease in pediatric ALCL. Leukemia. 2009;**23**(2):400-402

[26] Benharroch D et al. ALK-positive lymphoma: A single disease with a broad spectrum of morphology. Blood. 1998;**91**(6):2076-2084

[27] Lamant L et al. Prognostic impact of morphologic and phenotypic features of childhood ALK-positive anaplastic large-cell lymphoma: Results of the ALCL99 study. Journal of Clinical Oncology. 2011;**29**(35):4669-4676

[28] Montes-Mojarro IA et al. The pathological Spectrum of systemic anaplastic large cell lymphoma (ALCL). Cancers (Basel). 2018 Apr 4;**10**(4). pii: E107. DOI: 10.3390/cancers10040107

[29] Malcolm TI et al. Challenging perspectives on the cellular origins of lymphoma. Open Biology. 2016 Sep;**6**(9). pii: 160232

[30] Malcolm TI et al. Anaplastic large cell lymphoma arises in thymocytes and requires transient TCR expression for thymic egress. Nature Communications. 2016;**7**:10087

[31] Youssif C et al. Genomic profiling of pediatric ALK-positive anaplastic large cell lymphoma: A Children's Cancer and Leukaemia Group Study. Genes, Chromosomes & Cancer. 2009;**48**(11):1018-1026

[32] Salaverria I et al. Genomic profiling reveals different genetic aberrations in systemic ALK-positive and ALK-negative anaplastic large cell lymphomas. British Journal of

Haematology. 2008;**140**(5):
516-526

[33] Duyster J, Bai RY, Morris SW. Translocations involving anaplastic lymphoma kinase (ALK). Oncogene. 2001;**20**(40):5623-5637

[34] Shiota M, Mori S. Anaplastic large cell lymphomas expressing the novel chimeric protein p80NPM/ALK: A distinct clinicopathologic entity. Leukemia. 1997;**11**(Suppl 3):538-540

[35] Crockett DK et al. Identification of NPM-ALK interacting proteins by tandem mass spectrometry. Oncogene. 2004;**23**(15):2617-2629

[36] Marzec M et al. Oncogenic tyrosine kinase NPM/ALK induces activation of the rapamycin-sensitive mTOR signaling pathway. Oncogene. 2007;**26**(38):5606-5614

[37] Marzec M et al. Oncogenic tyrosine kinase NPM/ALK induces activation of the MEK/ERK signaling pathway independently of c-Raf. Oncogene. 2007;**26**(6):813-821

[38] Turner SD et al. The NPM-ALK tyrosine kinase mimics TCR signalling pathways, inducing NFAT and AP-1 by RAS-dependent mechanisms. Cellular Signalling. 2007;**19**(4):740-747

[39] Turner SD et al. Vav-promoter regulated oncogenic fusion protein NPM-ALK in transgenic mice causes B-cell lymphomas with hyperactive Jun kinase. Oncogene. 2003;**22**(49):7750-7761

[40] Zamo A et al. Anaplastic lymphoma kinase (ALK) activates Stat3 and protects hematopoietic cells from cell death. Oncogene. 2002;**21**(7):1038-1047

[41] Bai RY et al. Nucleophosmin-anaplastic lymphoma kinase of large-cell anaplastic lymphoma is a constitutively active tyrosine kinase that utilizes phospholipase C-gamma to mediate its mitogenicity. Molecular and Cellular Biology. 1998;**18**(12):6951-6961

[42] Cui YX et al. NPM-ALK inhibits the p53 tumor suppressor pathway in an MDM2 and JNK-dependent manner. Blood. 2009;**113**(21):5217-5227

[43] Ambrogio C et al. NPM-ALK oncogenic tyrosine kinase controls T-cell identity by transcriptional regulation and epigenetic silencing in lymphoma cells. Cancer Research. 2009;**69**(22):8611-8619

[44] Marzec M et al. Oncogenic kinase NPM/ALK induces through STAT3 expression of immunosuppressive protein CD274 (PD-L1, B7-H1). Proceedings of the National Academy of Sciences of the United States of America. 2008;**105**(52):20852-20857

[45] Zhang Q et al. IL-2R common gamma-chain is epigenetically silenced by nucleophosphin-anaplastic lymphoma kinase (NPM-ALK) and acts as a tumor suppressor by targeting NPM-ALK. Proceedings of the National Academy of Sciences of the United States of America. 2011;**108**(29):11977-11982

[46] Zhang Q et al. STAT5A is epigenetically silenced by the tyrosine kinase NPM1-ALK and acts as a tumor suppressor by reciprocally inhibiting NPM1-ALK expression. Nature Medicine. 2007;**13**(11):1341-1348

[47] Zhang Q et al. STAT3 induces transcription of the DNA methyltransferase 1 gene (DNMT1) in malignant T lymphocytes. Blood. 2006;**108**(3):1058-1064

[48] McDonnell SR et al. Integrated phosphoproteomic and metabolomic profiling reveals NPM-ALK-mediated phosphorylation of PKM2 and metabolic reprogramming in

anaplastic large cell lymphoma. Blood. 2013;**122**(6):958-968

[49] Hassler MR et al. Insights into the pathogenesis of anaplastic large-cell lymphoma through genome-wide DNA methylation profiling. Cell Reports. 2016;**17**(2):596-608

[50] Merkel O et al. Identification of differential and functionally active miRNAs in both anaplastic lymphoma kinase (ALK)+ and ALK− anaplastic large-cell lymphoma. Proceedings of the National Academy of Sciences of the United States of America. 2010;**107**(37):16228-16233

[51] Bonzheim I et al. Anaplastic large cell lymphomas lack the expression of T-cell receptor molecules or molecules of proximal T-cell receptor signaling. Blood. 2004;**104**(10):3358-3360

[52] Marzec M et al. Malignant transformation of CD4+ T lymphocytes mediated by oncogenic kinase NPM/ALK recapitulates IL-2-induced cell signaling and gene expression reprogramming. Journal of Immunology. 2013;**191**(12):6200-6207

[53] Matsuyama H et al. miR-135b mediates NPM-ALK-driven oncogenicity and renders IL-17-producing immunophenotype to anaplastic large cell lymphoma. Blood. 2011;**118**(26):6881-6892

[54] Desjobert C et al. MiR-29a down-regulation in ALK-positive anaplastic large cell lymphomas contributes to apoptosis blockade through MCL-1 overexpression. Blood. 2011;**117**(24):6627-6637

[55] Dejean E et al. Hypoxia-microRNA-16 downregulation induces VEGF expression in anaplastic lymphoma kinase (ALK)-positive anaplastic large-cell lymphomas. Leukemia. 2011 Dec;**25**(12):1882-1890. DOI: 10.1038/leu.2011.168. Epub 2011 Jul 22

[56] Spaccarotella E et al. STAT3-mediated activation of microRNA cluster 17~92 promotes proliferation and survival of ALK-positive anaplastic large cell lymphoma. Haematologica. 2014;**99**(1):116-124

[57] Crescenzo R et al. Convergent mutations and kinase fusions lead to oncogenic STAT3 activation in anaplastic large cell lymphoma. Cancer Cell. 2015;**27**(4):516-532

[58] Feldman AL et al. Discovery of recurrent t(6;7)(p25.3;q32.3) translocations in ALK-negative anaplastic large cell lymphomas by massively parallel genomic sequencing. Blood. 2011;**117**(3):915-919

[59] Vasmatzis G et al. Genome-wide analysis reveals recurrent structural abnormalities of TP63 and other p53-related genes in peripheral T-cell lymphomas. Blood. 2012;**120**(11):2280-2289

[60] Scarfo I et al. Identification of a new subclass of ALK-negative ALCL expressing aberrant levels of ERBB4 transcripts. Blood. 2016;**127**(2): 221-232

[61] Merkel O et al. Oncogenic role of miR-155 in anaplastic large cell lymphoma lacking the t(2;5) translocation. The Journal of Pathology. 2015 Aug;**236**(4):445-456. DOI: 10.1002/path.4539. Epub 2015 Apr 27

[62] Steinhilber J et al. Next-generation sequencing identifies deregulation of microRNAs involved in both innate and adaptive immune response in ALK+ ALCL. PLoS One. 2015;**10**(2):e0117780

[63] Laginestra MA et al. Pathogenetic and diagnostic significance of microRNA deregulation in peripheral T-cell lymphoma not otherwise specified. Blood Cancer Journal. 2014;**4**:259

[64] Liu C et al. MicroRNA expression profiling identifies molecular signatures associated with anaplastic large cell lymphoma. Blood. 2013;**122**(12):2083-2092

[65] Piva R et al. Gene expression profiling uncovers molecular classifiers for the recognition of anaplastic large-cell lymphoma within peripheral T-cell neoplasms. Journal of Clinical Oncology. 2010;**28**(9):1583-1590

[66] Piccaluga PP et al. Molecular profiling improves classification and prognostication of nodal peripheral T-cell lymphomas: Results of a phase III diagnostic accuracy study. Journal of Clinical Oncology. 2013;**31**(24):3019-3025

[67] Agnelli L et al. Identification of a 3-gene model as a powerful diagnostic tool for the recognition of ALK-negative anaplastic large-cell lymphoma. Blood. 2012;**120**(6):1274-1281

[68] Iqbal J et al. Molecular signatures to improve diagnosis in peripheral T-cell lymphoma and prognostication in angioimmunoblastic T-cell lymphoma. Blood. 2010;**115**(5):1026-1036

[69] Boi M et al. PRDM1/BLIMP1 is commonly inactivated in anaplastic large T-cell lymphoma. Blood. 2013;**122**(15):2683-2693

[70] Keech JA Jr, Creech BJ. Anaplastic T-cell lymphoma in proximity to a saline-filled breast implant. Plastic and Reconstructive Surgery. 1997;**100**(2):554-555

[71] Administration, U.F.a.D. Anaplastic large cell lymphoma (ALCL) in women with breast implants: Preliminary findings and analyses. 2011. Available from: http://wayback.archive-it.org/7993/20171115053750/https:/www.fda.gov/MedicalDevices/ProductsandMedicalProcedures/ImplantsandProsthetics/BreastImplants/ucm239996.htm

[72] Ministere des affaires sociales, d.l.s.e.d.d.d.f., La France reste vigilante pour detecter rapidement les cas de lymphomes parmi les femmes porteuses d'implants mammaires. 2015

[73] Administration, U.F.a.D., Breast Implant-Associated Anaplastic Large Cell Lymphoma (BIA-ALCL). 2017

[74] Antonella C, Rosaria B, Marcella M. 22 cases of BIA-ALCL: Awareness and outcome tracking from the Italian Ministry of Health. Plastic and Reconstructive Surgery. 2017

[75] Johnson L et al. Breast implant associated anaplastic large cell lymphoma: The UK experience. Recommendations on its management and implications for informed consent. European Journal of Surgical Oncology. 2017;**43**(8):1393-1401

[76] de Jong D et al. Anaplastic large-cell lymphoma in women with breast implants. JAMA. 2008;**300**(17):2030-2035

[77] Laurent C et al. Breast implant-associated anaplastic large cell lymphoma: Two distinct clinicopathological variants with different outcomes. Annals of Oncology. 2016;**27**(2):306-314

[78] Clemens MW, Miranda RN. Coming of age: Breast implant-associated anaplastic large cell lymphoma after 18 years of investigation. Clinics in Plastic Surgery. 2015;**42**(4):605-613

[79] Doren EL et al. U.S. epidemiology of breast implant-associated anaplastic large cell lymphoma. Plastic and Reconstructive Surgery. 2017;**139**(5):1042-1050

[80] Srinivasa DR et al. Global adverse event reports of breast implant-associated ALCL: An international review of 40 government authority databases. Plastic and Reconstructive Surgery. 2017;**139**(5):1029-1039

[81] Ramos-Gallardo G et al. Is Latin America Ready to Identify Anaplastic Large Cell Lymphoma in Breast Implants Patients? Regional Encounter during the National Plastic Surgery Meeting in Cancun. Mexico: Aesthetic Plast Surg; 2018

[82] McGuire P, Reisman NR, Murphy DK. Risk factor analysis for capsular contracture, malposition, and late Seroma in subjects receiving Natrelle 410 form-stable silicone breast implants. Plastic and Reconstructive Surgery. 2017;**139**(1):1-9

[83] de Boer M et al. Breast implants and the risk of anaplastic large-cell lymphoma in the breast. JAMA Oncology. 2018;**4**:335-341

[84] Loch-Wilkinson A et al. Breast implant-associated anaplastic large cell lymphoma in Australia and New Zealand: High-surface-area textured implants are associated with increased risk. Plastic and Reconstructive Surgery. 2017;**140**(4):645-654

[85] Clemens MW, Horwitz SM. NCCN consensus guidelines for the diagnosis and management of breast implant-associated anaplastic large cell lymphoma. Aesthetic Surgery Journal. 2017;**37**(3):285-289

[86] Clemens MW et al. Complete surgical excision is essential for the management of patients with breast implant-associated anaplastic large-cell lymphoma. Journal of Clinical Oncology. 2016;**34**(2):160-168

[87] Ye X et al. Anaplastic large cell lymphoma (ALCL) and breast implants: Breaking down the evidence. Mutation Research, Reviews in Mutation Research. 2014;**762**:123-132

[88] Lechner MG et al. Survival signals and targets for therapy in breast implant-associated ALK—Anaplastic large cell lymphoma. Clinical Cancer Research. 2012;**18**(17):4549-4559

[89] Kadin ME et al. Biomarkers provide clues to early events in the pathogenesis of breast implant-associated anaplastic large cell lymphoma. Aesthetic Surgery Journal. 2016;**36**(7):773-781

[90] Kadin ME et al. IL-13 is produced by tumor cells in breast implant associated anaplastic large cell lymphoma: Implications for pathogenesis. Human Pathology. 2018 Aug;**78**:54-62. DOI: 10.1016/j.humpath.2018.04.007. Epub 2018 Apr 22

[91] Blombery P et al. Whole exome sequencing reveals activating JAK1 and STAT3 mutations in breast implant-associated anaplastic large cell lymphoma anaplastic large cell lymphoma. Haematologica. 2016;**101**(9):e387-e390

[92] Di Napoli A et al. Targeted next generation sequencing of breast implant-associated anaplastic large cell lymphoma reveals mutations in JAK/STAT signalling pathway genes, TP53 and DNMT3A. British Journal of Haematology. 2018;**180**(5):741-744

[93] Bekkenk MW et al. Primary and secondary cutaneous CD30(+) lymphoproliferative disorders: A report from the Dutch cutaneous lymphoma group on the long-term follow-up data of 219 patients and guidelines for diagnosis and treatment. Blood. 2000;**95**(12):3653-3661

[94] Liu HL et al. CD30+ cutaneous lymphoproliferative disorders: The Stanford experience in lymphomatoid

papulosis and primary cutaneous anaplastic large cell lymphoma. Journal of the American Academy of Dermatology. 2003;**49**(6): 1049-1058

[95] Kempf W et al. EORTC, ISCL, and USCLC consensus recommendations for the treatment of primary cutaneous CD30-positive lymphoproliferative disorders: Lymphomatoid papulosis and primary cutaneous anaplastic large-cell lymphoma. Blood. 2011;**118**(15):4024-4035

[96] Krishnan J, Tomaszewski MM, Kao GF. Primary cutaneous CD30-positive anaplastic large cell lymphoma. Report of 27 cases. Journal of Cutaneous Pathology. 1993;**20**(3):193-202

[97] Kiran T et al. The significance of MUM1/IRF4 protein expression and IRF4 translocation of CD30(+) cutaneous T-cell lymphoproliferative disorders: A study of 53 cases. Leukemia Research. 2013;**37**(4):396-400

[98] Geller S et al. ALK-positive primary cutaneous anaplastic large cell lymphoma: A case report and review of the literature. International Journal of Dermatology. 2018;**57**(5):515-520

[99] Wada DA et al. Specificity of IRF4 translocations for primary cutaneous anaplastic large cell lymphoma: A multicenter study of 204 skin biopsies. Modern Pathology. 2011;**24**(4):596-605

[100] Pham-Ledard A et al. IRF4 gene rearrangements define a subgroup of CD30-positive cutaneous T-cell lymphoma: A study of 54 cases. The Journal of Investigative Dermatology. 2010;**130**(3):816-825

[101] Feldman AL et al. Recurrent translocations involving the IRF4 oncogene locus in peripheral T-cell lymphomas. Leukemia. 2009;**23**(3):574-580

[102] Szuhai K et al. Array-CGH analysis of cutaneous anaplastic large cell lymphoma. Methods in Molecular Biology. 2013;**973**:197-212

[103] Benner MF et al. Primary cutaneous anaplastic large cell lymphoma shows a distinct miRNA expression profile and reveals differences from tumor-stage mycosis fungoides. Experimental Dermatology. 2012;**21**(8):632-634

[104] Garner R et al. Long-term disease control of refractory anaplastic large cell lymphoma with vinblastine. Journal of Pediatric Hematology/Oncology. 2009;**31**(2):145-147

[105] Brugieres L et al. Single-drug vinblastine as salvage treatment for refractory or relapsed anaplastic large-cell lymphoma: A report from the French Society of Pediatric Oncology. Journal of Clinical Oncology. 2009;**27**(30):5056-5061

[106] Cederleuf H et al. The addition of etoposide to CHOP is associated with improved outcome in ALK+ adult anaplastic large cell lymphoma: A Nordic Lymphoma Group study. British Journal of Haematology. 2017;**178**(5):739-746

[107] Alderuccio JP et al. Frontline brentuximab vedotin in breast implant-associated anaplastic large-cell lymphoma. Clinical Case Reports. 2018;**6**(4):634-637

[108] Melchers RC et al. Evaluation of treatment results in multifocal primary cutaneous anaplastic large cell lymphoma: Report of the Dutch Cutaneous Lymphoma Group. The British Journal of Dermatology. 2018 Sep;**179**(3):724-731. DOI: 10.1111/bjd.16501. Epub 2018 Jun 21

[109] Melchers RC et al. Recommendations for the optimal radiation dose in patients with

primary cutaneous anaplastic large cell lymphoma: A report of the Dutch cutaneous lymphoma group. International Journal of Radiation Oncology, Biology, Physics. 2017;**99**(5):1279-1285

[110] Christensen JG et al. Cytoreductive antitumor activity of PF-2341066, a novel inhibitor of anaplastic lymphoma kinase and c-Met, in experimental models of anaplastic large-cell lymphoma. Molecular Cancer Therapeutics. 2007;**6**(12 Pt 1): 3314-3322

[111] Mosse YP et al. Safety and activity of crizotinib for paediatric patients with refractory solid tumours or anaplastic large-cell lymphoma: A Children's Oncology Group phase 1 consortium study. The Lancet Oncology. 2013;**14**(6):472-480

[112] Mosse YP et al. Targeting ALK with Crizotinib in pediatric anaplastic large cell lymphoma and inflammatory myofibroblastic tumor: A Children's oncology group study. Journal of Clinical Oncology. 2017;**35**(28):3215-3221

[113] Gambacorti-Passerini C, Mussolin L, Brugieres L. Abrupt relapse of ALK-positive lymphoma after discontinuation of Crizotinib. The New England Journal of Medicine. 2016;**374**(1):95-96

[114] Senter PD, Sievers EL. The discovery and development of brentuximab vedotin for use in relapsed Hodgkin lymphoma and systemic anaplastic large cell lymphoma. Nature Biotechnology. 2012;**30**(7):631-637

[115] Nielson C et al. Loss of CD30 expression in anaplastic large cell lymphoma following brentuximab therapy. Journal of Drugs in Dermatology. 2016;**15**(7): 894-895

[116] Arai H et al. ALK-negative anaplastic large cell lymphoma with loss of CD30 expression during treatment with brentuximab vedotin. Rinshō Ketsueki. 2016;**57**(5):634-637

[117] Pro B et al. Brentuximab vedotin (SGN-35) in patients with relapsed or refractory systemic anaplastic large-cell lymphoma: Results of a phase II study. Journal of Clinical Oncology. 2012;**30**(18):2190-2196

[118] Prince HM et al. Brentuximab vedotin or physician's choice in CD30-positive cutaneous T-cell lymphoma (ALCANZA): An international, open-label, randomised, phase 3, multicentre trial. Lancet. 2017;**390**(10094):555-566

[119] Pro B et al. Five-year results of brentuximab vedotin in patients with relapsed or refractory systemic anaplastic large cell lymphoma. Blood. 2017;**130**(25):2709-2717

[120] Laimer D et al. PDGFR blockade is a rational and effective therapy for NPM-ALK-driven lymphomas. Nature Medicine. 2012;**18**(11):1699-1704

[121] Chen J et al. Cytokine receptor signaling is required for the survival of ALK− anaplastic large cell lymphoma, even in the presence of JAK1/STAT3 mutations. Proceedings of the National Academy of Sciences of the United States of America. 2017;**114**(15):3975-3980

[122] Chiarle R et al. The anaplastic lymphoma kinase is an effective oncoantigen for lymphoma vaccination. Nature Medicine. 2008;**14**(6): 676-680

[123] Pulford K et al. Detection of anaplastic lymphoma kinase (ALK) and nucleolar protein nucleophosmin (NPM)-ALK proteins in normal and neoplastic cells with the

monoclonal antibody ALK1. Blood. 1997;**89**(4):1394-1404

[124] Moti N et al. Anaplastic large cell lymphoma-propagating cells are detectable by side population analysis and possess an expression profile reflective of a primitive origin. Oncogene. 2015 Apr 2;**34**(14):1843-1852. DOI: 10.1038/onc.2014.112. Epub 2014 May 12

[125] Laurent C et al. Circulating t(2;5)-positive cells can be detected in cord blood of healthy newborns. Leukemia. 2012;**26**(1):188-190

[126] Kasprzycka M et al. Nucleophosmin/anaplastic lymphoma kinase (NPM/ALK) oncoprotein induces the T regulatory cell phenotype by activating STAT3. Proceedings of the National Academy of Sciences of the United States of America. 2006;**103**(26):9964-9969

[127] Schleussner N et al. The AP-1-BATF and -BATF3 module is essential for growth, survival and TH17/ILC3 skewing of anaplastic large cell lymphoma. Leukemia. 2018 Sep;**32**(9):1994-2007. DOI: 10.1038/s41375-018-0045-9. Epub 2018 Mar 28

[128] Pearson JD et al. NPM-ALK and the JunB transcription factor regulate the expression of cytotoxic molecules in ALK-positive, anaplastic large cell lymphoma. International Journal of Clinical and Experimental Pathology. 2011;**4**(2):124-133

[129] Tripathi SK, Lahesmaa R. Transcriptional and epigenetic regulation of T-helper lineage specification. Immunological Reviews. 2014;**261**(1):62-83

[130] Lamant L et al. Cutaneous presentation of ALK-positive anaplastic large cell lymphoma following insect bites: Evidence for an association in five cases. Haematologica. 2010;**95**(3):449-455

[131] Piccaluga PP et al. Anaplastic lymphoma kinase expression as a marker of malignancy. Application to a case of anaplastic large cell lymphoma with huge granulomatous reaction. Haematologica. 2000;**85**(9):978-981

[132] Hu H et al. Bacterial biofilm infection detected in breast implant-associated anaplastic large-cell lymphoma. Plastic and Reconstructive Surgery. 2016;**137**(6):1659-1669

[133] Knorr F et al. Blood cytokine concentrations in pediatric patients with anaplastic lymphoma kinase-positive anaplastic large cell lymphoma. Haematologica. 2018;**103**(3):477-485

[134] Hernandez L et al. Diversity of genomic breakpoints in TFG-ALK translocations in anaplastic large cell lymphomas: Identification of a new TFG-ALK(XL) chimeric gene with transforming activity. The American Journal of Pathology. 2002;**160**(4):1487-1494

[135] Hernandez L et al. TRK-fused gene (TFG) is a new partner of ALK in anaplastic large cell lymphoma producing two structurally different TFG-ALK translocations. Blood. 1999;**94**(9):3265-3268

[136] Lamant L et al. A new fusion gene TPM3-ALK in anaplastic large cell lymphoma created by a (1;2)(q25;p23) translocation. Blood. 1999;**93**(9):3088-3095

[137] Wlodarska I et al. The cryptic inv(2)(p23q35) defines a new molecular genetic subtype of ALK-positive anaplastic large-cell lymphoma. Blood. 1998;**92**(8):2688-2695

[138] Ma Z et al. Inv(2)(p23q35) in anaplastic large-cell lymphoma induces

constitutive anaplastic lymphoma kinase (ALK) tyrosine kinase activation by fusion to ATIC, an enzyme involved in purine nucleotide biosynthesis. Blood. 2000;**95**(6):2144-2149

[139] Tort F et al. Molecular characterization of a new ALK translocation involving moesin (MSN-ALK) in anaplastic large cell lymphoma. Laboratory Investigation. 2001;**81**(3):419-426

[140] Cools J et al. Identification of novel fusion partners of ALK, the anaplastic lymphoma kinase, in anaplastic large-cell lymphoma and inflammatory myofibroblastic tumor. Genes, Chromosomes & Cancer. 2002;**34**(4):354-362

[141] Touriol C et al. Further demonstration of the diversity of chromosomal changes involving 2p23 in ALK-positive lymphoma: 2 cases expressing ALK kinase fused to CLTCL (clathrin chain polypeptide-like). Blood. 2000;**95**(10):3204-3207

[142] Lamant L et al. Non-muscle myosin heavy chain (MYH9): A new partner fused to ALK in anaplastic large cell lymphoma. Genes, Chromosomes & Cancer. 2003;**37**(4):427-432

[143] Lawrence B et al. TPM3-ALK and TPM4-ALK oncogenes in inflammatory myofibroblastic tumors. The American Journal of Pathology. 2000;**157**(2):377-384

[144] van, der Krogt JA et al. Anaplastic lymphoma kinase-positive anaplastic large cell lymphoma with the variant RNF213-, ATIC- and TPM3-ALK fusions is characterized by copy number gain of the rearranged ALK gene. Haematologica. 2017;**102**(9):1605-1616

Chapter 4

Extranodal T/NK Lymphomas

Silvana Novelli

Abstract

Extranodal T/NK lymphomas comprise infrequent and highly aggressive entities such as extranodal NK/T-cell lymphoma nasal type, enteropathy-associated T-cell lymphoma, monomorphic epitheliotropic intestinal T-cell lymphoma, intestinal T-cell lymphoma NOS, and hepatosplenic T-cell lymphoma. Except for NK/T lymphoma nasal type, there is scarce evidence to support a specific therapeutic regimen in first line and relapse. As the only potentially curative therapy is allogeneic hematopoietic stem cell transplantation, it should be assessed in relapsing/refractory NK/T lymphoma nasal type and in the first line after remission in the other extranodal NK/T lymphomas.

Keywords: extranodal lymphoma, NK/T-cell lymphoma, NK lymphoma, hepatosplenic

1. Introduction

In this chapter, the majority of extranodal T/NK lymphomas will be discussed proportionally to the amount of available evidence and its clinical relevance. The 2016 WHO classification [1] includes the following entities: extranodal NK/T-cell lymphoma nasal type, enteropathy-associated T-cell lymphoma, monomorphic epitheliotropic intestinal T-cell lymphoma, intestinal T-cell lymphoma NOS, and hepatosplenic T-cell lymphoma. In general, these are very infrequent and aggressive lymphomas, being the most prevalent the extranodal NK/T-cell lymphoma, nasal type. The current classification separates enteropathy-associated T-cell lymphoma from monomorphic epitheliotropic intestinal T-cell lymphoma in two different entities; in this way, intestinal T-cell lymphoma NOS remains a category to place unclassifiable histologies. Recent advances in gene expression profiling have allowed identify genes and proteins with potential role in pathogenesis. Collaboration between different centers is showing promising results that will surely modify and improve current treatments and prognosis. It will also help to increase the evidence in the new classification categories.

2. Extranodal NK/T-cell lymphoma, nasal type (ENKL)

2.1 General features

Natural killer (NK) neoplasias are divided into extranodal NK/T, nasal type, and NK aggressive leukemia. The "nasal type" distinction is explained because there is a predominant affection of nasal zone, nasopharynx, and upper respiratory airways (60–90% of cases). The "extra-nasal" type also exists but is infrequent; it affects non-nasal areas such as the skin, testicles, intestines, and muscles [2].

Several works have tried to identify biologic differences between both clinical manifestations but it has not been possible. The "extra-nasal" variant has a worse outcome; patients frequently present with B symptoms, advanced stages, hemophagocytosis, and cytopenias.

Unlike Asia and Latin America, ENKL is infrequent in our media representing approximately 2% of non-Hodgkin lymphomas [3].

2.2 Etiology

Epstein-Barr virus (EBV) is an important feature of ENKL [4]. More than 90% of reported cases were positive for EBNA-1 and EBER-1. EBV is present in an episomal form not integrated into the host DNA, with type II latency [5, 6].

2.3 Diagnosis

At the morphological level, angiocentric and angio-invasive infiltrates composed of small-medium-sized atypical lymphocytes with irregular nuclei and immunoblasts are evident. There is a variable infiltration of plasma cells and, to a lesser extent, of eosinophils and histiocytes. The presence of extensive necrosis is frequent.

By immunohistochemistry, the tumor NK cells can have two lines of origin:

NK line (65–75% of cases): CD2 (+), CD3-ε (+) cytoplasmic, CD56 (+/−), CD94 (+), cytotoxic markers (TIA, GZM-B, perforin) (+), and TCR-β (BF1) (−).

True T-line (25–35% of cases): CD2 (+), CD3-ε (+), CD5 (+), CD8 (+/−), TCR-β (BF1) (+), CD56 (−/+), and cytotoxic markers (+).

EBV is detected in almost all cases by in situ hybridization (EBER) and by Southern blot. The latent EBV membrane protein has a variable expression, so it is not advisable to detect the virus [7].

Early chromosomal examinations recognized del(6)(q21q25) as a repetitive chromosomal anomaly in ENKL. In view of investigations of 6q, including gene expression profiling (GEP), PRDM1, FOXO3, and PTPRK were recognized as putative tumor suppressor genes. A high expression of genes of cytotoxic molecules such as granzyme H and deregulation of the NF-κB, AKT, and JAK-STAT3 pathways were also present in ENKL. Half of the patients have mutations in *FAS* and <50% in *TP53*. *DDX3X* and *BCL6* are also mutated; the former was more frequently mutated in men and was associated with poor survival [8].

2.4 Staging and prognosis

Because the prognosis is different between the "nasal" and the "extranasal" variants, techniques to detect occult disease become clinically important.

It is advisable to use PET/CT since it has shown greater sensitivity. In those cases where there is evidence of involvement of the central nervous system, it is necessary to consider complementing the study with magnetic resonance imaging (MRI) [9, 10].

Bone marrow biopsy is part of staging and cannot yet be replaced by the extensive use of PET/CT in this entity [11].

The staging should be performed according to Ann Arbor since most clinical trials have established it that way. However, TNM staging is also widely used since it offers the advantage of better assessing tumor size and infiltration of adjacent organs and tissues of the localized stage [12].

The ENKL prognostic index includes both stage and other variables. This index is fundamental for decision-making [13].

The ENKL index punctuates the presence of "B" symptoms, Ann Arbor stage ≥III, LDH ≥1 × upper normal limit, and regional lymph nodes (N1-N3, not M1) involvement

Risk group	Number of factors	% 5-year OS	RR of death
Group 1	0	81	1
Group 2	1	64	1.8
Group 3	2	34	4.1
Group 4	3–4	7	13.6

OS, overall survival; RR, relative risk.

Table 1.
Survival and relative risk of death.

according to the TNM staging system. Every point increases the relative of death and impairs survival (see **Table 1**).

The viral quantification of EBV is useful to assess the tumor burden. Negative loads have a better prognosis than cases with low EBV load (<1000 copies/ml in plasma or <100 copies/mcg of mononuclear cell DNA) and that of high load. It is also useful to monitor the response to therapy. Therefore, it should be done whenever possible [14, 15].

2.5 Treatment

The treatment is planned according to the stage and the risk.

In patients with stages I–II and low risk, radiotherapy (≥54 Gy) is the best option. It has not been observed that adding chemotherapy improves the prognosis [2, 16, 17].

If we focus on cases with stages I–II, but intermediate risk and high risk, it has been shown that the best option is the combination of chemotherapy and radiotherapy.

In the JCOG0211 study, radiotherapy (50 Gy) and three cycles of dexamethasone, etoposide, ifosfamide, and carboplatin (DeVIC) were administered. The overall survival (OS) at 2 years was 78% (95% CI, 57–89%). It was compared with a historical control of patients treated only with radiotherapy (OS 45%). The overall response rate was 81% (77% complete response, CR) [18].

Another study showed similar results. Radiotherapy (40–52.8 Gy) and cisplatin 30 mg/m^2 weekly followed by three cycles of VIPD (etoposide 100 mg/m^2 days 1–3, ifosfamide 1200 mg/m^2 days 1–3, cisplatin 33 mg/m^2 days 1–3, and dexamethasone 40 mg days 1–4). The progression-free survival (PFS) and the OS estimated at 3 years were 85 and 86%, respectively [19].

ENKL is associated with a high expression of P glycoprotein that confers resistance to most anthracycline-based regimens. For this reason, non-dependent glycoprotein-P schemes have been designed.

The regimens that have demonstrated greater efficacy are based on L-asparaginase. However, they are associated with a high toxicity.

Also for stages IE–IIE (all risk groups), the DICE–L-asparaginase chemotherapy with radiotherapy (45 Gy) after four cycles vs. radiotherapy alone has been tested The CR rate was higher for patients in the sequential radiotherapy group (90.9%) than in the radiotherapy group (77.8%; p = 0.124). PFS and OS at 5 years after diagnosis were significantly higher for patients in the chemo-radiotherapy group (PFS: 89%; OS: 82%) than in the radiotherapy group (PFS: 49%, $p < 0.001$; OS: 49%, $p < 0.001$) [20].

In advanced stages, the treatment must take into account the functional status of the patient.

If the patient's general condition allows it (ECOG 0–2) and the patient is a candidate for an autologous hematopoietic stem cell transplant (ASCT), the first-line therapy will be the SMILE scheme followed by TASP (dexamethasone: 40 mg EV or oral, days

2–4; methotrexate: 2000 mg/m^2 EV, day 1; ifosfamide: 1500 mg/m^2 EV, days 2–4; *E. coli* L-asparaginase: 6000 U/m^2 EV, days 8, 10, 12, 14, 16, 18, and 20; etoposide: 100 mg/m^2 EV, days 2–4).

The overall response rate (ORR) and the complete responses after 2 cycles were 79% (90% CI, 65–89%) and 45%, respectively. Approximately half of the patients received an ASCT.

However, in those in the first line, the ORR was higher (86%), with CR of 69%. These responses were maintained in 90% of patients during follow-up. The OS at 1 year was 55% (95% CI, 38–69%). On the other hand, grade 4 neutropenia occurred in 92% of the cases [21, 22].

Another option for this high-risk group is the L-asparaginase, methotrexate, and dexamethasone (AspaMetDex) chemotherapy. In a phase 2 trial, it reported a CR rate of 61% after three cycles. Further results are needed to confirm the efficacy of this regimen [23].

In those patients with poor general condition and/or those who do not want to receive an ASCT, the management must be palliative or investigational since the prognosis is unfortunate.

However, there is evidence that the "sandwich" scheme of GELOX (gemcitabine, oxaliplatin, and L-asparaginase) and radiotherapy after at least two cycles of GELOX offers good results and acceptable toxicities in IE–IIE stages. The ORR was 96.3%, with CR of 74.1%. The OS and PFS at 2 years were both 86% [24, 25].

In relapse, if patients are tributary to treatment and have not received the SMILE scheme, this will become the second line based on the results described above. However, if the patient has been refractory to the SMILE scheme, the alternatives are also investigational and with scarce evidence.

There is a retrospective study with the GELOX scheme. The ORR was 40% (20% CR). Those who achieved CR (two received ASCT and maintenance with L-asparaginase) were disease free for 7 months [26].

Regarding ASCT and allogeneic stem cell transplantation (alloSCT), there is less evidence of its role in high risk and/or advanced stage ENKL.

There is a prospective study in the pre-L-asparaginase era which included 16 ENKL cases. Nine cases received an ASCT in first or second CR and the remaining in progression. The OS at 2 years was 71.3% (first to second CR) and 25.8%, respectively [27].

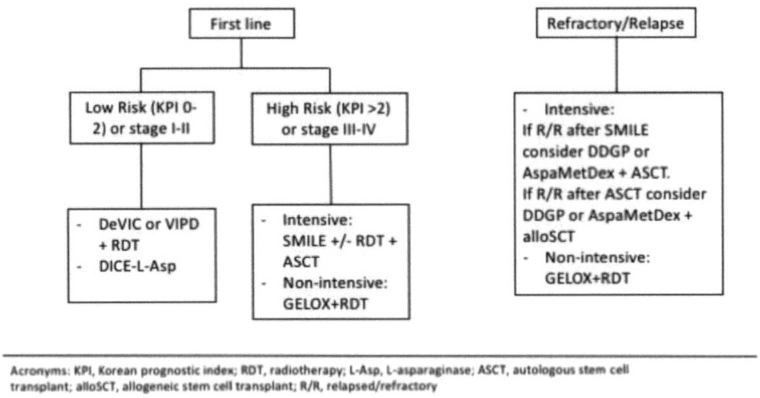

Figure 1.
Proposed treatments for extranodal NK/T-cell lymphoma, nasal type NK/T. KPI, Korean prognostic index; RDT, radiotherapy; L-Asp, L-asparaginase; ASCT, autologous stem cell transplant; alloSCT, allogeneic stem cell transplant; R/R, relapsed/refractory.

A registry study that includes 18 cases of patients who received an alloSCT demonstrated a PFS and OS at 5 years of 51 and 57%, respectively. Therefore, it becomes an alternative in very selected patients [28] (**Figure 1**).

New therapies, but not approved yet, are showing promising results. The most important results are those results obtained from the use of check point inhibitors (nivolumab and pembrolizumab). ORR oscillated between 57 and 100% but phase II trials are missing to confirm these results [29–31].

3. Enteropathy-associated T-cell lymphoma (EATL)

3.1 General features

The EATL currently refers exclusively to previous type I EATL and is clearly associated with celiac disease (CD) and occurs more frequently in patients of Northern European origin. Dermatitis herpetiformis and hyposplenism may be associated. Patients who are diagnosed at a higher age of celiac disease have a higher risk of having an LTAE and proper management with a gluten-free diet effectively prevents its development [32, 33].

The most affected regions are the jejunum or ileum and are usually diagnosed after a resection for an acute abdomen. Patients have a rapid deterioration of their general condition despite strictly following the diet.

Refractory celiac disease (RCD) is the precursor lesion. It is defined by histological changes associated with enteropathy in cases with strict diet for >12 months or severe and persistent symptoms that require a clinical intervention regardless of the duration of the strict diet. There is a sub-classification, RCD type I, if the intraepithelial lymphocytes show a normal phenotype and constitute a polyclonal population, and RCD type II, if the intraepithelial lymphocytes immunophenotype is aberrant and clonal products are detected on TCR gene rearrangement analysis [34].

Loss of heterozygosity at 9p21, involving CDKN2A/B locus, was detected in more than 50% of cases with EATL. Loss of 17p12-p13.2 (TP53) was reported in 23%, but a high frequency of aberrant nuclear p53 expression (75%) suggested alternate means of deregulation of this tumor suppressor. Surprisingly, there are more new findings in terms of etiology in the monomorphic epitheliotropic intestinal T-cell lymphoma, and this will be further revised.

3.2 Diagnosis

Endoscopic findings show one or multiple ulcerated intestinal masses or large exophytic masses. At the serological level, tissue anti-transglutaminase IgA and anti-endomysial IgA are the most sensitive and specific tests. The typing of HLA-DQ in search of the alleles that predispose to CD (DQ2/DQ8) is part of the diagnosis [35].

Histologically, EATL is characterized by a non-monomorphic infiltrate of cells with CD3 (+), CD7 (+), CD103 (+), cytotoxic proteins (+) CD8 (−/+), TCR-β (+/−), CD4 (−), CD5 (−), CD56 (−), and CD30 focally (+) in a subset of cases. Adjacent intraepithelial lymphocytes also have an aberrant immunophenotype CD3 (+), CD5 (−), CD8 (−), CD4 (−), and cytotoxic proteins (−).

At the cytogenetic level, gains of 1q and 5q are observed [36].

3.3 Staging and prognosis

Staging will be carried out with the Lugano system [37] (see **Table 2**) Diagnostic tests include a CT scan, an endoscopic study, and a bone marrow biopsy. The index

Stage I	Tumor confined to GI tract. Single primary site or multiple, non-contiguous lesions.	
Stage II	Tumor extending into abdomen from primary GI site.	Nodal involvement II_1 local (paragastric in cases of gastric lymphoma and para-intestinal for intestinal lymphoma) II_2 distant (mesenteric in the case of an intestinal primary, otherwise; para-aortic para-caval, pelvic, inguinal).
Stage IIE	Penetration of serosa to involve adjacent organs or tissues (enumerate actual site of involvement, e.g., $IIE_{pancreas}$, $IIE_{large\ intestine}$).	
Where there is both nodal involvement and penetration to involve adjacent organs, stage should be denoted using both a subscript ($_1$ or $_2$) and E, e.g., $II_1E_{pancreas}$.		
Stage IV	Disseminated extranodal involvement, or, a GI tract lesion with supra-diaphragmatic nodal involvement.	

Table 2.
Lugano staging system for gastrointestinal tract lymphoma.

that best defined prognosis of the EATL is the prognostic index used for peripheral T lymphomas (IPI) [38].

3.4 Treatment

Because at the time of diagnosis the patient is usually in advanced stages and have a poor nutritional status, therapeutic success is scarce.

Surgery plays an important role in reducing tumor burden and decreasing perforations or bleeding during chemotherapy, but on the other hand, it can delay the onset of chemotherapy [39, 40].

The most used chemotherapy is the CHOP scheme. Only 50% of patients will be able to receive chemotherapy, and of these, only 50% will complete it. Of those who complete chemotherapy, 35–40% will achieve a complete remission of the lymphoma. The median duration of the response is approximately 6 months [41].

In those patients who are candidates to receive an ASCT in first remission, it is advisable to do it following the EBMT recommendations [42]. In the most recent study of the EBMT registry, 31 cases of patients with EATL were identified. With a median of 46 months of follow-up, the SLP and the OS at 4 years were 54–59%, respectively [43].

Refractory patients are unlikely to benefit from a second line of chemotherapy. No superiority of any regimen has been demonstrated, so it is advisable to follow usual schemes in the center of origin [44].

4. Monomorphic epitheliotropic intestinal T-cell lymphoma (MEITL)

4.1 General features

The MEITL is the intestinal lymphoma that was previously classified as EATL type II. Because it has shown both clinical and biological differences with the EATL, it has been constituted as a new entity. It is not associated with celiac disease and has a greater incidence in Asian and Hispanic populations. Its frequency is 10–15% of intestinal T lymphomas.

4.2 Diagnosis

The tumor is composed of a monomorphic infiltrate. The immunophenotype is CD3 (+), CD8 (+), CD56 (+), TCR-β (+), CD4 (−).

In exceptional cases, TCR-γδ (+) has been demonstrated. Adjacent intraepithelial lymphocytes show an aberrant immunophenotype.

One way to differentiate it from other NK/T and EATL lymphomas is the positivity for the megakaryocyte-associated tyrosine kinase (MATK).

At the cytogenetic level, gains are observed in MYC (locus 8q24) [45].

The *staging and prognosis* will be carried out in the same way as for the EATL.

4.3 Treatment

There are no clinical trials that allow favoring one treatment regimen over another. However, there are retrospective studies where it is confirmed that the anthracycline regimens are the most used (72%). The overall response rate was 46% (CR 38%) [46].

Recently, the potential effect of pralatrexate has been reported in a relapsed patient after anthracycline containing regimen [47] and also the addition of PEG-asparaginase to EPOCH regimen in a non-responding patient [48].

The recommendations to perform an autologous transplant in the first remission are the same as in the EATL following the EBMT experience and recommendation for T-cell neoplasia [42, 49].

5. Hepatosplenic T-cell lymphoma (HSTL)

5.1 General features

HSTL is a rare entity. It represents 1% of non-Hodgkin's lymphoma and 3% of T-lymphoma. Survival at 5 years does not exceed 7%; therefore, it has a poor clinical prognosis [50].

The etiology is unclear; however, it is postulated that chronic stimulation in patients with immune deficiencies or immune dysregulation could be important. Twenty percent of cases occur in young patients with some degree of immunosuppression (posttransplant, under treatment of leukemia). It has also been associated with the use of TNFα and immunomodulators in patients with inflammatory bowel disease and arthritis [51, 52].

5.2 Diagnosis

It is characterized by the proliferation of malignant T cells of medium size in the hepatic sinusoids, in the red pulp of the spleen, and in the bone marrow. The immunophenotype of the tumor cell is CD4−, CD8− (CD8+ alginates), CD2+, CD3+, CD42, CD52, CD76, and CD82. The TCR is usually gamma-delta, although there are cases described alpha-beta. The detected cytogenetic anomalies include isochromosome 7q and trisomy 8 [53].

Recently, the genetic basis of HSTL was described using whole exome sequencing. Some chromatin-modifying genes (INO80, SETD2, and ARID1B) were commonly mutated in HSTL; there are frequent mutations in STAT5B (31%), STAT3 (9%), and PIK3CD (9%) and less frequent events in EZH2, KRAS, and TP53. SETD2 that works as a tumor suppressor gene was the most frequently silenced gene [54]. To further determine the pathogenesis, a multicenter group performed an array-based

DNA methylation profiling and identified eight genes consistently hypermethylated (BCL11B, CXCR6, CD5, GIMAP7, SEPT9, LTA, UBAC2, and UXS1) and four genes hypomethylated (ADARB1, NR1H3, NFIC, and ST3GAL3) [55].

5.3 Staging and prognosis

Staging is performed with the Ann Arbor system. A specific prognostic index for this lymphoma has not been described because of its low frequency.

5.4 Treatment

The most used treatments are CHOP and hyper-CVAD. The cases that respond can go directly to autologous or allogeneic transplant.

Other regimens described in a retrospective study (n = 14) have been ICE and IVAC in first line and also in rescue after CHOP. While it is a small series, the authors emphasize that the use of more intensive schemes followed by precursor transplant hematopoietic agents could improve efficacy data [56].

The relapse-free time and the OS post alloSCT are 18 and 68 months, respectively. The relapse-free time and the OS at 3 years are 42 and 56%, respectively. In this way, it is the only treatment that offers some probability of healing [57].

Author details

Silvana Novelli[1,2]

1 Hematology Department, Hospital de la Santa Creu i Sant Pau, Biomedical Research Institute (IIB Sant-Pau), Autonomous University of Barcelona, Spain

2 José Carreras Leukemia Research Institute, Autonomous University of Barcelona, Spain

*Address all correspondence to: snovelli@santpau.cat

References

[1] Swerdlow SH. World Health Organization; International Agency for Research on Cancer. WHO Classification of Tumours of Haematopoietic and Lymphoid Tissues. Revised 4th edition. Lyon: International Agency for Research on Cancer; 2017

[2] Au W et al. ENKL nasal or ex-nasal. Blood. 2016;**113**(17):3931-3938

[3] William BM, Armitage JO. International analysis of the frequency and outcomes of NK/T-cell lymphomas. Best Practice & Research. Clinical Haematology. 2013;**26**(1):23-32

[4] Harabuchi Y, Yamanaka N, Kataura A, Imai S, Kinoshita T, Osato T. Epstein-Barr virus in nasal T-cell lymphomas in patients with lethal midline granuloma. Lancet. 1990;**335**(8682):128-130

[5] Van Gorp J et al. Epstein-Barr virus in nasal T-cell lymphomas (polymorphic reticulosis/midline malignant reticulosis) in Western China. The Journal of Pathology. 1994;**173**(2):81-87

[6] Chan JK et al. Detection of Epstein-Barr viral RNA in malignant lymphomas of the upper aerodigestive tract. The American Journal of Surgical Pathology. 1994;**18**(9):938-946

[7] Medeiros LJ, Miranda RN. Diagnostic Pathology. Lymph Nodes Extranodal Lymphomas. Second edition. Philadelphia, PA: Elsevier; 2018

[8] Yamaguchi M, Oguchi M, Suzuki R. Extranodal NK/T-cell lymphoma: Updates in biology and management strategies. Best Practice & Research. Clinical Haematology. 2018;**31**(3):315-321

[9] Kim SJ et al. Risk stratification on the basis of Deauville score on PET-CT and the presence of Epstein-Barr virus DNA after completion of primary treatment for extranodal natural killer/T-cell lymphoma, nasal type: A multicentre, retrospective analysis. Lancet Haematology. 2015;**2**(2):e66-e74

[10] Guan H, Huang Y, Wen W, Xu M, Zan Q, Zhang Z. Primary central nervous system extranodal NK/T-cell lymphoma, nasal type: Case report and review of the literature. Journal of Neuro-Oncology. 2011;**103**(2):387-391

[11] Barrington SF et al. Role of imaging in the staging and response assessment of lymphoma: Consensus of the International Conference on Malignant Lymphomas imaging Working Group. Journal of Clinical Oncology. 2014;**32**(27):3048-3058

[12] Yan Z et al. A TNM staging system for nasal NK/T-cell lymphoma. PLoS One. 2015;**10**(6):1-17

[13] Lee J et al. Extranodal natural killer T-cell lymphoma, nasal-type: A prognostic model from a retrospective multicenter study. Journal of Clinical Oncology. 2006;**24**(4):612-618

[14] Au W, Pang A, Choy C, Chim C, Kwong Y, Dc W. Quantification of circulating Epstein-Barr virus (EBV) DNA in the diagnosis and monitoring of natural killer cell and EBV-positive lymphomas in immunocompetent patients. Blood. 2004;**104**(1):243-249

[15] Suzuki R et al. Prospective measurement of Epstein-Barr virus-DNA in plasma and peripheral blood mononuclear cells of extranodal NK/T-cell lymphoma, nasal type. Blood. Dec 1 2011;**118**(23):6018-6022

[16] Yang Y et al. Risk-adapted therapy for early-stage extranodal nasal-type NK/T-cell lymphoma: analysis from a multicenter study Blood. 2015;**126**:1424-1432

[17] Juan Huang M et al. Early or up-front radiotherapy improved

survival of localized extranodal NK/T-cell lymphoma, nasal-type in the upper aerodigestive tract. International Journal of Radiation Oncology, Biology, Physics. 2008;**70**(1):166-174

[18] Yamaguchi M et al. Phase I/II study of concurrent chemoradiotherapy for localized nasal natural killer/T-cell lymphoma: Japan Clinical Oncology Group Study JCOG0211. Journal of Clinical Oncology. 2009;**27**(33):5594-5600

[19] Kim SJ et al. Phase II trial of concurrent radiation and weekly cisplatin followed by VIPD chemotherapy in newly diagnosed, stage IE to IIE, nasal, extranodal NK/T-cell lymphoma: Consortium for improving survival of lymphoma study. Journal of Clinical Oncology. 2009;**27**(35):6027-6032

[20] Dong L-H et al. Sequential DICE combined with L-asparaginase chemotherapy followed by involved field radiation in newly diagnosed, stage IE to IIE, nasal and extranodal NK/T-cell lymphoma. Leukemia & Lymphoma. 2016;**57**(7):1600-1606

[21] Yamaguchi M et al. Phase II study of SMILE chemotherapy for newly diagnosed stage IV, relapsed, or refractory extranodal natural killer (NK)/T-cell lymphoma, nasal type: The NK-cell tumor study group study. Journal of Clinical Oncology. 2011;**29**(33):4410-4416

[22] Kwong Y et al. SMILE for natural killer/T-cell lymphoma: Analysis of safety and efficacy from the Asia Lymphoma Study Group. Blood. 2012;**120**(15):2973-2981

[23] Jaccard A et al. Efficacy of L-asparaginase with methotrexate and dexamethasone (AspaMetDex regimen) in patients with refractory or relapsing extranodal NK/T-cell lymphoma, a phase 2 study. Blood. 2011;**117**(6):1834-1839

[24] Wang L et al. First-line combination of gemcitabine, oxaliplatin, and L-asparaginase (GELOX) followed by involved-field radiation therapy for patients with stage IE/IIE extranodal natural killer/T-cell lymphoma. Cancer. 2013;**119**(2):348-355

[25] Wang H et al. Comparison of gemcitabine, oxaliplatin and L-asparaginase and etoposide, vincristine, doxorubicin, cyclophosphamide and prednisone as first-line chemotherapy in patients with stage IE to IIE extranodal natural killer/T-cell lymphoma: A multicenter retrospective study. Leukemia & Lymphoma. 2015;**56**(4):971-977

[26] Ahn HK et al. Gemcitabine alone and/or containing chemotherapy is efficient in refractory or relapsed NK/T-cell lymphoma. Investigational New Drugs. 2013;**31**(2):469-472

[27] Kim HJ et al. High-dose chemotherapy with autologous stem cell transplantation in extranodal NK/T-cell lymphoma: A retrospective comparison with non-transplantation cases. Bone Marrow Transplantation. 2006;**37**(9):819-824

[28] Tse E et al. Allogeneic haematopoietic SCT for natural killer/T-cell lymphoma: A multicentre analysis from the Asia Lymphoma Study Group. Bone Marrow Transplantation. 2014;**49**(7):902-906

[29] Lai J, Xu P, Jiang X, Zhou S, Liu A. Successful treatment with anti-programmed-death-1 antibody in a relapsed natural killer/T-cell lymphoma patient with multi-line resistance: A case report. BMC Cancer. 2017;**17**(1):507

[30] Li X et al. Activity of pembrolizumab in relapsed/refractory NK/T-cell lymphoma. Journal of Hematology & Oncology. 2018;**11**(1):15

[31] Chan TSY, Li J, Loong F, Khong P-L, Tse E, Kwong Y-L. PD1

blockade with low-dose nivolumab in NK/T cell lymphoma failing L-asparaginase: Efficacy and safety. Annals of Hematology. 2018;**97**(1):193-196

[32] Silano M et al. Effect of a gluten-free diet on the risk of enteropathy-associated T-cell lymphoma in celiac disease. Digestive Diseases and Sciences. 2008;**53**(4):972-976

[33] Lebwohl B et al. Mucosal healing and risk for lymphoproliferative malignancy in celiac disease: A population-based cohort study. Annals of Internal Medicine. 2013;**159**(3):169-175

[34] Chander U, Leeman-Neill RJ, Bhagat G. Pathogenesis of enteropathy-associated t cell lymphoma. Current Hematologic Malignancy Reports. 2018;**13**(4):308-317

[35] Stamnaes J, Sollid LM. Celiac disease: Autoimmunity in response to food antigen. Seminars in Immunology. 2015;**27**(5):343-352

[36] deLeeuw RJ et al. Whole-genome analysis and HLA genotyping of enteropathy-type T-cell lymphoma reveals 2 distinct lymphoma subtypes. Gastroenterology. 2007;**132**(5):1902-1911

[37] Rohatiner A et al. Report on a workshop convened to discuss the pathological and staging classifications of gastrointestinal tract lymphoma. Annals of Oncology. 1994;**5**(5):397-400

[38] Delabie J et al. Enteropathy-associated T-cell lymphoma: Clinical and histological findings from the international peripheral T-cell lymphoma project. Blood. 2011;**118**(1):148-155

[39] Nijeboer P et al. Treatment response in enteropathy associated T-cell lymphoma; survival in a large multicenter cohort. American Journal of Hematology. 2015;**90**(6):493-498

[40] Novakovic BJ, Novakovic S, Frkovic-Grazio S. A single-center report on clinical features and treatment response in patients with intestinal T cell non-Hodgkin's lymphomas. Oncology Reports. 2006;**16**(1):191-195

[41] Di Sabatino A, Biagi F, Gobbi PG, Corazza GR. How I treat enteropathy-associated T-cell lymphoma. Blood. 2012;**119**(11):2458-2468

[42] Sureda A et al. Indications for allo- and auto-SCT for haematological diseases, solid tumours and immune disorders: Current practice in Europe. Bone Marrow Transplantation. 2015;**50**(8):1037-1056, 2015

[43] Jantunen E et al. Autologous stem cell transplantation in adult patients with peripheral T-cell lymphoma: A nation-wide survey. Bone Marrow Transplantation. 2004;**33**(4):405-410

[44] Raderer M et al. Second line chemotherapy in patients with enteropathy-associated T cell lymphoma: A retrospective single center analysis. Annals of Hematology. 2012;**91**(1):57-61

[45] Chen Y, Tan S-Y, Petersson BF, Khor YM, Gopalakrishnan SK, Tan D. Occult recurrence of monomorphic epitheliotropic intestinal T-cell lymphoma and the role of MATK gene expression in diagnosis. Hematological Oncology. 2017;**35**(4):852-855

[46] Tse E et al. Type II enteropathy-associated T-cell lymphoma: A multicenter analysis from the Asia Lymphoma Study Group. American Journal of Hematology. 2012;**87**(7):663-668

[47] Tabata R, Tabata C, Okamura M, Takei Y, Ohshima K. Successful treatment of monomorphic epitheliotropic intestinal T cell lymphoma with pralatrexate. Annals of Hematology. May 2019;**98**(5):1301-1303

[48] Gentille C, Qin Q, Barbieri A, Ravi PS, Iyer S. Use of PEG-asparaginase in monomorphic epitheliotropic intestinal T-cell lymphoma, a disease with diagnostic and therapeutic challenges. ecancermedicalscience. 2017;**11**:771

[49] Jantunen E, Boumendil A, Finel H. Autologous stem cell transplantation for enteropathy-associated T-cell lymphoma: A retrospective study by the EBMT. Blood. 2013;**121**(13):2529-2532

[50] Vose JM, Neumann M, Harris ME. International peripheral T-cell and natural killer/T-cell lymphoma study: Pathology findings and clinical outcomes international T-cell lymphoma project. Journal of Clinical Oncology. 2008;**26**(25):4124-4130

[51] Weidmann E. Hepatosplenic T cell lymphoma. A review on 45 cases since the first report describing the disease as a distinct lymphoma entity in 1990. Leukemia. 2000;**14**(6):991-997

[52] Parakkal D, Sifuentes H, Semer R, Ehrenpreis ED. Hepatosplenic T-cell lymphoma in patients receiving TNF-α inhibitor therapy: Expanding the groups at risk. European Journal of Gastroenterology & Hepatology. 2011;**23**(12):1150-1156

[53] Calvaruso M et al. Challenges and new prospects in hepatosplenic γδ T-cell lymphoma. Leukemia & Lymphoma. 2014;**55**:1-9

[54] McKinney M et al. The genetic basis of hepatosplenic T-cell lymphoma. Cancer Discovery. 2017;7(4):369-379

[55] Bergmann AK et al. DNA methylation profiling identifies candidate genes for the pathogenesis of hepatosplenic T-cell lymphoma. Haematologica. 2018;**2018**:196196

[56] Voss MH et al. Intensive induction chemotherapy followed by early high-dose therapy and hematopoietic stem cell transplantation results in improved outcome for patients with hepatosplenic T-cell lymphoma: A single institution experience. Clinical Lymphoma, Myeloma & Leukemia. 2013;**13**(1):8-14

[57] Rashidi A, Cashen AF. Outcomes of allogeneic stem cell transplantation in hepatosplenic T-cell lymphoma. Blood Cancer Journal. 2015;**5**:e318

Chapter 5

Gamma-Delta T-cell Lymphoma: An Overview

Preethi Ramachandran, Alok Aggarwal and Jen Chin Wang

Abstract

Gamma-delta T-cell lymphomas are very rare and aggressive T-cell neoplasms with complex heterogenicity and diagnostic complexity. Gamma-delta T lymphocytes originate from CD4– CD8– (double negative) thymocytes in the bone marrow and are distinct from alpha beta subtype. Four entities of gamma-delta lymphomas recognized by 2016 WHO classification of lymphoid neoplasms include: hepatosplenic Tγδ lymphoma (HSγδTL), primary cutaneous gamma-delta TCL (PCTCL), monomorphic epitheliotropic intestinal T-cell lymphoma (MEITL) and large granular lymphocytic leukemias (T-LGL). Extensive literature search based on small case series and case reports identifies few more subtypes of gamma-delta T-lymphomas which were not previously classified by World Health Organization. There remains a critical gap in our understanding of the subtypes of gamma-delta T-cell lymphomas and a lack of updated summarization. In this review, we summarize in detail on the classification, biology, heterogenicity, diagnosis, clinical behavior and treatment options of these rare but clinically important entities.

Keywords: gamma-delta T-cell, T cell lymphoma, non-Hodgkin lymphoma, T-cell receptor, hepatosplenic T cell lymphoma

1. Introduction

T/NK (natural killer) cell lymphomas are uncommon lymphomas accounting for about 6% of all non-Hodgkin lymphoma (NHL). B-cell lymphomas account for the majority being 80% and Hodgkin lymphoma accounts for 7% of NHLs in the United States according to the Surveillance, Epidemiology, and End Results program (SEER) over a 10-year period from 1997 till 2006 [1]. According to the updated 2016 revision of World Health Organization Classification (WHO) of T-cell lymphoid neoplasms, there are about 27 types of mature T and NK cell neoplasms. Amongst all types, gamma-delta T-cell lymphoma (γδ-TCL) accounts for only <1% of lymphoid tumors [2].

T lymphocytes recognize antigens through T-cell receptors (TCRs). TCRs are polypeptide heterodimers which mostly constitutes α and β chains and rarely γ and δ chains. Alpha-beta T cells (Tαβ) constitute 95% of all T cells while gamma-delta T cells (Tγδ) make up only a small proportion accounting to <5% of all circulating lymphocytes. Majority of lymphoid tissues are made of αβ T cells than γδ subtype. Gamma-delta (γδ) subtype shows selective tropism for the red pulp of the spleen, mucosal tissues, gastrointestinal epithelial tissues, skin and rarely lymphoid tissue. Hence the γδ T cells have a higher representation of about 30% in some epithelial-rich tissues, such as intestine and sinusoidal red pulp of the spleen [3]. Most of the T-cell lymphomas have alpha-beta TCRs while only 5% of the T-NHL's have gamma-delta TCRs [4].

2. T-cell receptor

T-cell receptors are complex membrane proteins which are found on the surface of T lymphocytes through which the T cells recognize the antigens. The antigens are recognized as peptides linked to major histocompatibility complex (MHC) molecules [5]. T lymphocytes recognize antigens through T cell receptors (TCRs). TCRs are polypeptide heterodimers composed of two different protein chains. These two chains mostly consist of alpha (α) chain and a beta (β) chain in 95% of the cases whereas in 5%, these chains are composed of gamma and delta (γ/δ) chains. Alpha and beta chains are encoded by T-cell receptor alpha (TRA) at 14q11.2 and T-cell receptor beta (TRB) gene at 7q34. The gamma and delta chains are encoded by T cell receptor gamma locus (TRG) (7p14) and T cell receptor delta locus (TRD) (14q11.2) genes respectively [6]. TRαβ recognizes processed antigens presented by MHC proteins whereas TR γδ recognizes non-peptide antigens.

After the T cell lineage commitment is made, the progenitors make their first lineage decision to be either αβ or γδ. CD4– CD8– (double negative) thymocytes rearrange three out of four TCR loci: Tcrb, Tcrg, and Tcrd. The cells which are arrested

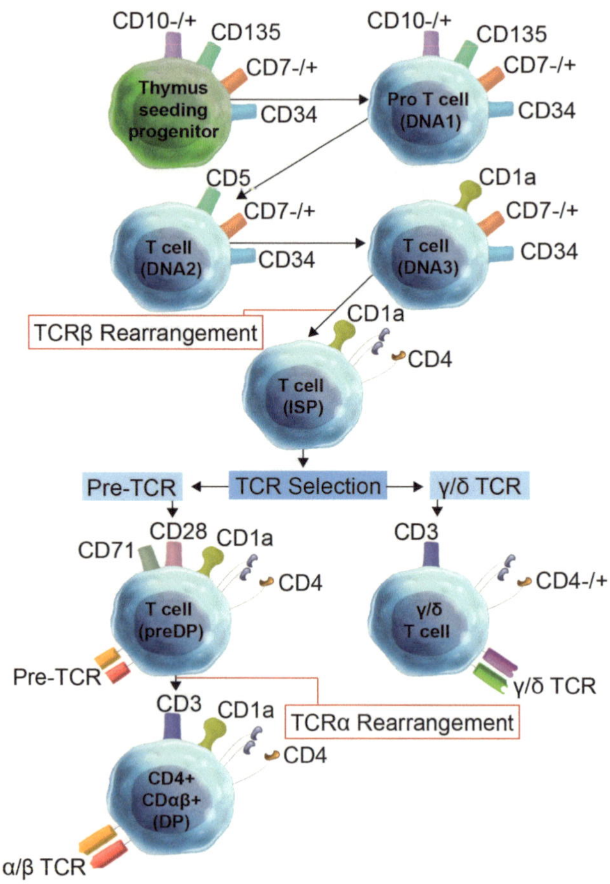

Figure 1.
Illustration of T cell development.

in proliferation at this stage require expression of TCR to re-enter the cell cycle. If there is a success in an in-frame Tcrb rearrangement, TCRβ is expressed which forms a complex with the germline-encoded pre-TCRα (pTα) chain [3]. Increased upregulation of CD4 and CD8 receptors along with increased proliferation occurs when this complex is expressed. Tcrq is silenced and Tcra rearrangement starts thus resulting in excision of Tcrd locus. CD4+ CD8+ [double positive (DP)] thymocytes express TCRαβ and further differentiate into CD4+ or CD8+ lineages when there is a rearrangement of T cell receptor alpha chain (Tcra). Progression through the DP stage is believed to be a hallmark of αβ lineage commitment. Thymocyte progenitors which have a rearrangement of Tcrg and Tcrd will express γδTCR at the cell surface. These cells also undergo increased proliferation but tend to avoid going through the DP stage thus arriving at the periphery as CD4− CD8− (or, more rarely, with CD4− CD8+ or CD4+ CD8−) cells. Hence the lineage toward αβ or γδ is based on the progression towards the DP stage [7]. See **Figure 1** for illustration of T-cell development.

3. Gamma-delta T cells

Gamma-delta T lymphocytes originate from CD4− CD8− (double negative) thymocytes in the bone marrow and do not need recognition by the major histocompatibility complex [8]. The antigenic stimulus that activates these subtype of cells is unknown. These lymphocytes have properties of cytotoxicity, phagocytosis [9, 10] and also play a major role in both innate immunity and non-specific immune responses [11–13].

There are two variable receptor regions within the T cell receptor in gamma delta T cells which divide them into two subtypes—Vdelta1 and Vdelta2 gamma delta T-cells [14, 15]. These two subtypes further differ in their phenotypes and the regions of distribution

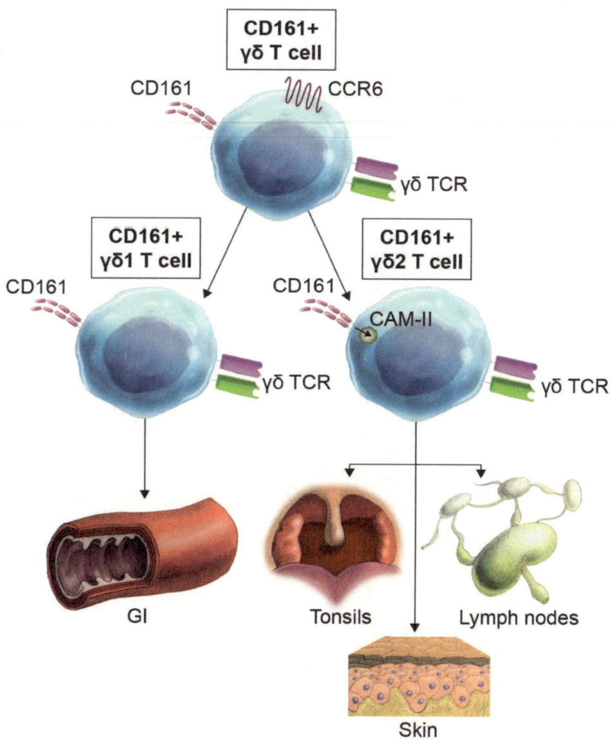

Figure 2.
Illustration γδ of T cell function and the roles of specific subsets. Vdelta1 T cells are more predominant in gastrointestinal tract and Vdelta2 cells in skin, lymphoid tissue and tonsils.

within the body. While Vdelta1 T cells are more predominant in gastrointestinal tract, Vdelta2 T cells are seen mostly in skin, lymphoid tissue and tonsils. See **Figure 2** for illustration of summary of γδ T-cell functions and the roles of specific subsets.

4. WHO 2016 revised classification

Gamma-delta T-cell lymphomas constitute a very rare and aggressive subtype of lymphomas with a very poor prognosis [16]. The gamma delta T-cell lymphomas were classified into two groups in 2008 by the World Health Organization (WHO) as hepatosplenic Tγδ cell lymphoma (HSγδTL) and primary cutaneous TCL (PCTCL) [17]. In 2016, the WHO classification of T Tγδ cell lymphoma added few more subgroups.

As per 2016 revision of the WHO classification of lymphoid neoplasms, the four recognized entities of Tγδ cell lymphoma identified includes,

1. Hepatosplenic Tγδ cell lymphoma (HSγδTL)
2. Primary cutaneous gamma delta TCL (PCTCL)
    a. Aggressive variant
    b. Mycosis fungoides like (Indolent variant)
3. Monomorphic epitheliotropic intestinal TCL (MEITL)
4. Gamma-delta large granular lymphocytic leukemias (T-LGL)

Although the WHO classification is helpful in defining the subtypes of lymphomas, there are other rare variants of gamma-delta T-cell lymphomas in literature in the form of case reports which still remains unclassifiable. Based on an extensive literature search, we classify gamma delta T-cell lymphomas into the five subtypes as illustrated in **Table 1**.

1. Hepatosplenic Tγδ cell lymphoma (HSγδTL)
2. Primary cutaneous gamma-delta T-cell lymphoma (PCTCL)
    a. Aggressive variant
    b. Mycosis fungoides like (indolent variant)
    c. Subcutaneous panniculitis-like
3. Mucosal gamma-delta T-cell lymphoma
    a. Gastrointestinal
    b. Nasal
    c. Pulmonary
    d. Laryngeal
4. Gamma-delta T-LGL
5. Nodal gamma-delta T-cell lymphoma

Types	Age	Incidence	Gender	Median survival	Subtypes	EBV association	Clinical features	Treatment
Hepatosplenic Gamma delta T-cell lymphoma	Young adults (35 yrs)	<1%	Male	<2 yrs	None	Yes	Cytopenia, Infiltration of liver, spleen and BM. LN rare	CHOP like regimen Allogenic stem cell transplant Relapsed cases - Bendamustine, bortezomib, lenlidomide, vorinostat.
Primary cutaneous gamma delta T-cell lymphoma	Adults	<1%	None	15 months	Aggressive Mycosis fungoides-like Subcutaneous panniculitis-like	No	Papule, plaque or nodule with ulceration and overlying epidermal necrosis	CHOP-like regimen Steoid, MTX, UV radiation, Bexarotene
Mucosal Gamma delta T-cell lymphoma	>48 yrs	NK	None	1-1.5 yrs	Gastrointestina Nasal Pulmonary Laryngeal	Yes	HSM, Nasal destruction GI perforation LN and BM involvement rare	CHOP like regimen Allogenic stem cell transplantation
Gamma delta T-LGL	45-75 yrs	2-3%	None	Indolent	None	Yes, in few cases	Cytopenia, splenomegaly, BM involved	Steroids, MTX, cyclosporine, cyclophosphamide, fludarabine, pentostatin
Nodal gamma delta T-Cell lymphoma	NK	<2%	NK	<1 yr	None	yes	LN, BM infiltration, HSM	CHOP-like regimen Allogenic stem cell transplant

Table 1.
Classification of gamma-delta T-cell lymphomas.

5. Gene expression profiling of gamma delta lymphoma

Research studies have shown that the different molecular profiling exists between γδTCL and αβTCL as well as the existence of a distinct molecular signature in hepatosplenic gamma delta T cell lymphoma.

Kana Miyazaki et al. analyzed RNA from seven patients with gamma delta T cell lymphoma (four hepatosplenic, one cutaneous, one intestinal and one thyroidal) and 27 patients with alpha beta T cell lymphoma (11 peripheral TCL unspecified, 15 angioimmunoblastic TCL and one hepatosplenic) using oligonucleotide microarrays. Based on the genetic analysis, they classified hepatosplenic γδTCL as a single cluster, whereas other γδTCL were more heterogeneous and were scattered within the αβ distribution. Gene expression profiles were compared between γδTCL and αβTCLs, using 291 genes. Webgestalt analysis using Gene Ontology (GO) hierarchies for categorizing functional gene groups and Kyoto Encyclopedia of gene and genomes (KEGG) pathway was used for identifying signaling pathways. They concluded that five in γδTCL and 20 in αβTCL gene groups were expressed under the GO category and three γδTCL pathways and one αβTCL pathway were found to be altered in KEGG-signaling analyses. These studies concluded that no signature genes were shared between γδTCL and αβTCL thereby confirming different functional profiling between them. Genes encoding KIRs and killer cell lectin-like receptors were seen in four out of five γδTCL enriched GO categories and two out of three KEGG signaling pathways, thus becoming a very important marker in differentiating γδTCL from αβTCL [18].

6. Types of gamma delta T-cell lymphoma

6.1 Hepatosplenic Tγδ cell lymphoma (HSγδTL)

Hepatosplenic gamma delta T cell lymphoma is one of the types of gamma delta T-cell lymphoma with an aggressive clinical course and poor overall survival rates [19]. The average length of survival seems to be <16 months [20]. The unique feature of this type of T cell lymphoma is the extranodal involvement with a specific sinusoidal pattern of infiltration of the liver, red pulp of spleen and bone marrow [21]. It also has unique immunophenotypical and chromosomal abnormality distinguishing it from other subtypes of gamma delta T cell lymphomas [22].

6.1.1 Incidence and etiology

Hepatosplenic Tγδ cell lymphoma seems to be predominantly a disease of young age mostly affecting teenage and young adults. They represent <5% of all peripheral T cell lymphomas. Males are affected more than females with a male/female ratio of 10/1. Although chronic antigenic stimulation and immune dysregulation seems to be likely causative factor in the evolution of this disorder [23], most of the cases (72%) of HSGDTCL occurs in patients with no underlying immunosuppression. Only around 18% of patients have underlying immunosuppression in the form of either previous organ transplants, chronic steroids use, inflammatory bowel disease, autoimmune disorders and hematological malignancies especially of acute myeloid leukemia, multiple myeloma, and Hodgkin lymphoma. About 10% of the patients have a history of previous treatment with immunosuppressive or biologics especially azathioprine and infliximab [24]. There are few cases reporting associations with Epstein-Barr Virus (EBV) and hepatitis B infections in the literature [25].

6.1.2 Pathology

The histopathological feature of HSGDTL includes monomorphous infiltration of medium-sized lymphocytes with a moderate amount of large pale basophilic cytoplasm [23, 26–28]. These cells have loosely condensed nuclear chromatin with small inconspicuous nucleoli. Spleen shows an involvement of sinuses of red pulp with atrophic white pulp. Involvement of liver is predominantly in the sinusoids. Bone marrow involvement occurs with predominantly intrasinusoidal distribution. An interstitial pattern of bone marrow involvement with a shift towards blastic cells are features of disease progression. Lymph node involvement is very rare.

Immunophenotypic origin is from double negative CD4− CD8− cells which show CD2+ CD3+ CD5− CD7+, TCRγδ+ [28, 29]. NK cell markers (DC16, CD56, CD57) may occasionally be expressed. They also show expression of cytotoxic granule-associated proteins such as TIA1 and granzyme M but are negative for granzyme B and perforin [22, 29]. A minority of variant forms of HSGDTL shows TCR αβ expression.

The most common cytogenetic abnormality seen in HSGDTL is isochromosome 7q abnormality [i(7q)]. Trisomy 8 and deletion of Y chromosome are other genetic abnormalities sometimes encountered. The primary cytogenetic event which occurs initially is i(7q) while the other genomic alteration occurs when the disease progresses [30–32].

6.1.3 Molecular genetics of HSGDTL

Although isochromosome 7q is the most common chromosomal abnormality detected so far in HSTL, recent genomic analysis by Julio Finalet Ferreiro et al. identified a rare variant aberration of ring 7 [r(7)], thereby narrowing down the critical 7p/7q regions and identifying the targeted genes. They did genomic and transcriptomic study of six i(7) (q10) and ring 7 [r(7)] cases of HSTL, thereby mapping the common deleted region (CDR) at 7p22.1p14.1 (34.88 Mb; 3,506,316–38,406,226 bp) and the common gained region (CGR) at 7q22.11q31.1 (38.77 Mb; 86,259,620–124,892,276 bp). They postulated that loss of 7p22.1p14.1 enhanced the expression of CHN2 (7p14.1)/b2-chimerin leading to downmodulation of the NFAT pathway thereby increasing proliferation. They also hypothesized that the multidrug resistance gene ABCB1, RUNDC3B, PPP1R9A have an increased expression with the amplification of 7q22.11q31.1, thereby providing a growth advantage for the tumor cells further increasing their intrinsic chemoresistance. They distinguished HSTL from other malignancies by identifying a set of 24 genes by doing gene expression profile of HSTL, including three located on chromosome 7 (CHN2, ABCB1, and PPP1R9A) [33].

McKinney et al. did detailed study on the whole exome sequencing of 68 HSTL cases and identified the commonly mutated genes including SETD2, INO80, and ARID1B in 62% of HSTL cases. Mutations were also identified in STAT5B (31%), STAT3 (9%), and PIK3CD (9%) which has targeted treatments currently. The most commonly silenced gene was found to be SETD (tumor suppressor gene). Cell survival in HSTL was linked to the mutations in STAT5B and PIK3CD which activates the critical signaling pathways [34].

6.1.4 Staging

Staging of HSGDTL is based on the physical examination, hematological and biochemical parameters, imaging studies including computed tomography (CT) and positron emission tomography (PET) scans, bone marrow biopsy and gastrointestinal tract examination. Experience of PET imaging in T cell lymphomas is anecdotal when compared to B cell lymphomas [35–37]. Ann-Arbor staging system is used for staging of HSGDTL like any other NHL [38]. As per this staging, HSGDTL is classified as stage IV disease commonly presenting with systemic symptoms, hepatosplenic involvement with rare occurrence of bulky disease.

6.1.5 Postulated cell of origin

HSGDTCL is believed to arise from the immature non-activated gamma-delta T cells (T$\gamma\delta$) of Vdelta1 subtype which are predominantly seen in the gastrointestinal tract [39–41].

6.1.6 Clinical presentation

HSGDTL is mainly a disease of young men affecting in their second or third decade of life [42]. Main presenting features include systemic symptoms, hepatosplenomegaly and the absence of lymphadenopathy. The presenting feature of HSGDTL as per literature review include cytopenia, splenomegaly, fever, weight loss, fatigue and easy bruising. Laboratory abnormality included anemia, thrombocytopenia, neutropenia, mildly elevated AST, ALT and alkaline phosphatase. Markedly elevated lactate dehydrogenase (LDH) is a frequently observed phenomenon. Fifty to 80% of cases can have peripheral neoplastic lymphocytes [20]. Very rarely can present with autoimmune hemolytic anemia [43]. Bone marrow involvement is very frequent at diagnosis [20, 44] Cytopenia is related to bone marrow infiltration, hypersplenism, and cytokine-induced hemophagocytic histiocytosis [45]. Re-appearance of thrombocytopenia is used as an indicator of relapse of disease in a patient who is in complete remission. Cutaneous and mediastinal involvement is very unusual. Presence of lymphadenopathy is very rare and would virtually rule out the possibility of HSGDTL.

6.1.7 Treatment and prognosis

There exists no consensus in the treatment of these lymphomas due to its rarity and limited possibility of prospective trials. Most commonly used treatment regimen is CHOP (cyclophosphamide, doxorubicin, vincristine, and prednisone) regimen with an acceptable response rate between 30 and 45%. But even with those who achieve complete remission, the median time to relapse remains around 4 months [22, 46, 47]. Few other treatment options previously tried includes corticosteroids, alkylating agents, anthracycline-containing agents like CHOP/HYPERCVAD regimen, purine analogs and cytarabine-cisplatin combination. Few cases have reported clinical response with alemtuzumab combined with purine analogs but no overall survival benefit was noted [48–50]. But this combination causes significant hematological toxicity causing deeper immunosuppression and the risk of infection reactivations.

Autologous and allogeneic stem cell transplantations have been used as a modality of treatment with good response. There are case reports which support bortezomib in combination with high dose CHOP chemotherapy followed by BEAM autograft as well as CHOP regimen followed by high dose methotrexate, high dose cyclophosphamide with subsequent autograft using conditioning regimen containing etoposide, ifosfamide, and ranimustine [51]. Allogeneic stem cell transplantation has previously been tried with encouraging results but at the expense of treatment-related mortality. Various myeloablative conditioning regimen has been tried usually including total body irradiation. Relapse-free interval has been shown to be between 12 and 58 months after treatment of aggressive disease with allogeneic transplant. Relapsed/refractory disease is usually resistant to conventional chemotherapy and there are previous case reports of successful second allogeneic transplant for patients who failed the first allograft [52]. Relapse of the disease is usually seen in the initially involved sites but lymphadenopathy is uncommon which signifies the homing of these neoplastic cells.

Treatment of relapsed/refractory disease with single agents like bevacizumab, vorinostat, lenalidomide, bortezomib, bendamustine and etoposide has been reported in single cases but no large case series data exist about their efficacy [53–59]. HSGDTL is a very aggressive disease which is resistant to most of the conventional chemotherapeutic agents. The median survival has been estimated to be <1 year for those treated with a CHOP-like regimen. Most of the patients do not live longer than 2 years [14]. Even though there is a lack of clear prognostic factors, data from small case series suggests male sex, lack of TCR rearrangements and failure of response has been shown to have negative outcomes [42]. New onset thrombocytopenia has been linked to the recurrence and severity of the disease in few cases [20].

6.2 Primary cutaneous gamma delta T-cell lymphoma (PCGD-TCL)

As per 2016 WHO classification of mature lymphoid, histiocytic and dendritic neoplasms, cutaneous T cell lymphomas are classified as subcutaneous panniculitis-like T cell lymphoma, mycosis fungoides (MF), Sezary syndrome, primary cutaneous gamma delta T cell lymphomas (PCGD-TCL), lymphoid polyposis, CD30+ primary cutaneous anaplastic large cell lymphoma, primary cutaneous CD8+ aggressive epidermotropic cytotoxic T cell lymphomas, primary cutaneous acral CD8+ T-cell lymphoma, primary cutaneous lymphomas, not otherwise classified (PCTL, NOS), extranodal nasal-type NK/T-cell lymphomas and primary cutaneous CD4+ small/medium T-cell lymphoproliferative disorder.

Primary cutaneous gamma delta T-cell lymphomas is a rare malignancy with a very aggressive course. There also exists rarer variants which have an indolent course as per few case reports [60]. Primary cutaneous gamma delta T-cell lymphomas have a preference for extremities and can present either as plaque, tumor or subcutaneous nodules. They do not exhibit EBV positivity and mostly have a mature cytotoxic phenotype.

6.2.1 Incidence and risk factors

PCGD-TCL accounts for <1% of all cutaneous TCLs [17]. It arises from clonal proliferation of cytotoxic gamma-delta T-cells in the skin. Mostly all cases are grouped as either mycosis fungoides-like or subcutaneous panniculitis-like cutaneous lymphomas. Generally, these mucocutaneous subtypes are not related to Epstein-Barr virus infections [61].

Chronic antigenic stimulation along with decreased immunity remains the underlying risk factor for developing this disease. Some of the other risk factors seem to be underlying autoimmunity, malignancy, viral hepatitis and other lymphoproliferative disorders.

6.2.2 Pathology

Histologically the infiltration patterns can involve epidermis, dermis and subcutaneous tissue. These patterns can be present separately or can be seen within the same lesion [23]. The presentation can be disseminated, necrotizing or ulcerative. Pathological features involve angioinvasion, angiodestruction, and necrosis. Epidermal involvement may vary from being mild epidermotrophic to a marked pagetoid variety [62]. In the subcutaneous panniculitis type, infiltration with medium to large neoplastic cells with clumped chromatin is seen around adipose tissues. Occasionally blastoid cells with prominent nucleoli are noted.

The neoplastic cells usually express CD2 and CD3 and are usually negative for CD4 and CD8. They also express CD7, CD56 and frequently are positive for cytotoxic proteins like TIA-1, granzyme B, and perforin. They do not express βF1.

TCRγ expression has also been reported in other primary cutaneous TCLs especially in mycosis fungoides and lymphomatoid papulosis. Even though these lymphomas are CD8 negative, few cases of CD8+ PCGD-TCLs have been reported [16].

6.2.3 Molecular genetics

Neoplastic cells always express TCRγ and TCRδ genetic rearrangements. They are also negative for EBV encoded RNA emphasizing that EBV infection does not play any role in their pathogenesis [23]. PCGD-TCLs show very complex cytogenetic alterations which include translocations involving breakpoints at 9p21, 14q11.2, 14q32.1 or 16q23.1. This suggests that the tumor evolvement is related to WWOX, TCL gene cluster, and BCL11B [63].

Other pathways involved in tumorigenesis includes pathways related to RAS, P13KT/MTOR, TP53 and MYC related signaling [26]. There are no characteristic mutations identified so far.

6.2.4 Staging

Staging involves a complete workup including hematological evaluation, biochemical evaluation, gastrointestinal evaluation, bone marrow biopsy, PET CT and/or computed tomography scans. Most commonly used staging system for PCGD-TCL is the International Society for Cutaneous Lymphoma/European Organization of Research and Treatment of Cancer (ISCL/EORTC) TNM classification system of cutaneous lymphoma other than mycosis fungoides and Sezary syndrome [64].

6.2.5 Clinical presentation

Most of the cases occur in older adults with a median age of 60 years. There seems to be no gender preference and both sexes are equally affected [65]. PCGD-TCL shows diffuse skin involvement with a predilection for extremities, thighs, and buttocks and spares the trunk. They may present either as a papule, plaque or nodule with ulceration and overlying epidermal necrosis. Few cases present as panniculitis either with dermal or subcutaneous infiltration [61].

In one of the study gamma delta cutaneous T-cell lymphomas have been shown to have a poor survival when compared with alpha-beta subtype. The median survival for the former was 15 months whereas it was 166 months for latter. It was also found that patients who had subcutaneous involvement had decreased survival (13 months) compared to those who had epidermotrophic or dermal involvement (29 months). Poor prognostic factors included gamma delta phenotype, subcutaneous involvement, and presentation as clinical tumors [16].

Most of the patients have B symptoms like fever, weight loss, and an elevated LDH. Hemophagocytic syndrome is more likely with panniculitis like presentation [61]. Although most of the cases of PCGD-TCL is aggressive, there are also cases which are indolent. This indolent variety has been described previously as "ketron-goodman type" presenting as verrucoid lesions [53]. Mucosal and extranodal dissemination mainly to GI tract and nasopharynx are seen [66–72]. Widespread dissemination is rare and involvement if spleen, liver and bone marrow are infrequent. Only very few cases have lymph node involvement [73]. Rare cases of metastasis to testis and central nervous system have been reported.

6.2.6 Treatment and prognosis

No standard treatment exists due to the rarity of this disease. Hence the treatment guidelines are mostly based on case reports. Most commonly used regimen remains to be doxorubicin-based regimen like CHOP. About 50% of the patients showed response but subsequently had a relapse of the disease with tumor progression and death. Steroids have been used with increased remission rate [74]. Low dose methotrexate and narrow-band ultraviolet radiation have also been used in few types of PCGDTL presenting as patch/plaque [75]. Bexarotene as a single agent and in combination was used as maintenance after CHOP-like regimen showing good response [76].

Due to the aggressive nature of the disease, autologous and allogeneic stem cell transplant has also been tried. In a small case series (n = 13) complete remission rate of 92% was achieved with stem cell transplant. But this study included alpha/beta phenotype as well which impairs the application of the results. The more indolent subtype remains responsive to steroids without the need for a more aggressive approach [60].

The overall prognosis seems to be very poor due to aggressive nature and chemotherapy resistance of these lymphomas. They have a median survival of 15 months and a 5-year overall survival is around 10% [16]. But the more indolent subtypes usually have slightly better prognosis when compared to aggressive subtype. Poor prognostic factors included subcutaneous involvement, age > 40 years, associated cytopenias, tumors expressing CD56, CD95 without expressing CD8, extensive ulcerated lesions at presentation, central nervous system (CNS) involvement and the presence of hemophagocytic syndrome as per the largest reported series [77, 78].

6.3 Mucosal gamma delta TCL

This type of lymphoma affects the mucosal tract lining nasopharynx, intestine, breast, larynx, lung, and testis indicating the homing of these γδ T-cells. These are very aggressive lymphomas and due to the rarity of the disease, information regarding the presentation and treatment is only from small case series.

6.3.1 Incidence and risk factors

Mucosal gamma-delta lymphoma is very rare aggressive tumor whose incidence cannot be predicted due to rarity and limited literature evidence. Chronic antigenic stimulation along with prolonged immune suppression seems to be a major risk factor in the development of this disease. Patients with underlying hypogammaglobulinemia, selective IgA deficiency, and T cell deficiency are more prone to develop this disease. In one of the case series, it was found that patients who developed nasal lymphoma had past history of chronic sinusitis. Similarly, pulmonary lymphomas developed in a background of opportunistic pulmonary infections. Gastric and intestinal lymphomas had a predisposing factor of *H. pylori* and coeliac sprue [26, 66, 79].

6.3.2 Pathology

Morphologically they are variable in nature presenting either as small to medium-sized cells or as large pleomorphic variants. Occasionally cells had abundant clear cytoplasm with irregular nuclei with condensed chromatin. Other features commonly seen include angioinvasion, angiocentrism, epitheliotropism and necrosis [42].

Most of them express TCRγδ (δTCR1+) but are negative for TCR αβ. They commonly express CD2 and CD3 but did not express CD4, CD8, and CD5. CD7 may be variable. CD56 is expressed mostly by nasal T-cell lymphomas and are infrequent in other types. Since the tumor arises from activated cytotoxic T cells, there is a positive expression for T cell intracellular antigen 1 (TIA1), granzyme B, and perforin. EBV association has been reported in nasal, laryngeal and gastrointestinal mucosal gamma-delta T-cell lymphoma. EBV-encoded latent membrane protein studied by immunohistochemistry is found positive in these variants [42].

6.3.3 Genetic abnormality

Neoplastic cells showed clonal γ chain rearrangement showing evidence of T cell lineage and clonality. They show positivity for EBV encoded RNA emphasizing that EBV infection does play a role in their pathogenesis. No other characteristic mutations have been identified so far.

6.3.4 Clinical presentation

Mucosal gamma-delta T-cell lymphomas usually have an aggressive course with high recurrence rate presenting both with a local and systemic disease. In one of the case series, the median age of the patient was 48 years. Nasal lymphomas present as destructive nasal lesions as well as nasal obstruction. Gastrointestinal lymphomas usually involve either localized or diffuse areas of the gut thereby presenting as peritonitis and perforation [66]. Most of the patients present with B symptoms but rarely have any lymphadenopathy or bone marrow involvement. Elevated LDH and hypogammaglobulinemia were observed in few cases [66].

6.3.5 Treatment and prognosis

Due to the rarity of the disease, no guidelines exist. Literature evidences are available for treatment with CHOP-like regimen and stem cell transplantation. Clinical outcome is mostly associated with short overall survival. Durable remission was seen only in few cases. In a small case series of 11 patients, most of the patients died within 1 year and only three had some durable response lasting more than a year [66].

6.4 Gamma delta T-LGL

Gamma-delta T-LGL represents 2–3% of all mature lymphocytic leukemia. Most of the T-LGL have αβ rearrangements and are positive for CD8, CD16, CD57. γδ T-cell large granular lymphocytic (T-LGL) is a very rare heterogeneous disorder of mature lymphocytes with unique morphology and an indolent clinical course. Although this variant is similar to the common T-LGL, some differences exist in clinical presentation, immunophenotype and organ involvement.

6.4.1 Incidence and risk factors

γδ T-LGL accounts for <5% of all T-LGLs. Usually, this type of lymphoma presents in patients >50 years old. Underlying immunosuppression is an associated risk factor for its development. Association with rheumatoid arthritis has been reported in about 20% of cases of γδ T-LGL and 25% of αβ T-LGL [80–82].

6.4.2 Pathology

Neoplastic cells can be infiltrated most commonly in bone marrow and spleen. When present in peripheral blood, they appear as large granular lymphocytes with azurophilic granules. Bone marrow involvement is characterized by lymphoid aggregates especially in the interstitial and intrasinusoidal areas [83]. Splenic involvement is characterized by infiltration of small lymphocytes with dense chromatin mostly concentrated in the red pulp rather than the white pulp [84, 85].

The neoplastic cells show positivity for pan T cell antigens CD2, CD3, and CD7. CD5 may be variable. They are usually CD8 positive and CD4 negative but cases with CD8 positivity has been reported previously [80, 81, 83, 86]. They show variable expression for CD16, CD56, and CD57. Cytotoxic markers like granzyme B and TIA-1 are seen in all cases. Flow cytometry usually shows positive expression for TCRγδ (δTCR1+) and is negative for TCR αβ. Immunohistochemical studies show TCRγ and negative for βF1 (marker for TCRβ).

6.4.3 Genetics

Neoplastic cells showed clonal γ chain rearrangement showing evidence of T cell lineage and clonality. Due to similar immunophenotype, especially of CD4-CD8– T-LGL with hepatosplenic gamma-delta T-cell lymphoma, further cytogenetic and FISH analysis need to be done to prove negativity for isochromosome 7q (i7q) [80, 83].

6.4.4 Clinical presentation

B symptom is common particularly with fever and fatigue predominating. The lab abnormality includes anemia, neutropenia, and thrombocytopenia with some cases presenting with increased severity. Not all patients present with lymphocytosis and occasionally lymphopenia is also observed. The peripheral smear shows large lymphocytes with prominent azurophilic granules in patients presenting with lymphocytosis. Splenomegaly is a common finding, but lymphadenopathy is rare. Bone marrow involvement is present mostly and shows predominantly an interstitial or less commonly intrasinusoidal pattern of infiltration. Associated autoimmune disorders like autoimmune hemolytic anemia (AIHA), immune thrombocytopenic purpura (ITP), rheumatoid disorder, pure red cell aplasia is also commonly observed [83].

6.4.5 Treatment and prognosis

The clinical course is mostly indolent. T-LGL generally is a chronic disorder with a good 10-year survival of 80% with around half of the patients not requiring any therapy [80, 81, 83, 87]. Spontaneous regression has been seen in few cases [88, 89]. The common reason for therapy remains to be low blood counts followed by hemolysis and splenomegaly. Several treatments like methotrexate, cyclophosphamide, cyclosporine, fludarabine, pentostatin either alone or in combination with steroids have been tried [90–93]. More resistant or advanced disease needs cytotoxic chemotherapy. Clinical course can be aggressive especially if they express CD56 antigen [94]. Splenectomy was also done as part of the treatment of ITP associated with this disorder.

6.5 Nodal gamma delta TCL

Nodal gamma delta TCL is a very rare subtype within gamma delta T-cell lymphomas. Very limited information is available in the literature due to the extreme rarity of this variant. So far only six cases of nodal gamma delta lymphomas have been reported. Usually, the presentation is in the form of disseminated nodal involvement.

6.5.1 Incidence and risk factors

Incidence difficult to predict due to the rarity of the disease. Chronic antigenic stimulation associated with immunosuppression plays a major role in the pathogenesis. Few case reports also suggest the role of EBV in lymphomagenesis.

6.5.2 Pathology

Neoplastic cells are very variable. They can present as a diffuse pleomorphic proliferation of small to medium-sized lymphoid cells with an irregular nucleus and moderate cytoplasm. They can also present as large pleomorphic cells or anaplastic or angioimmunoblastic like cells [42]. In one case report describing two cases of nodal gamma delta T-cell lymphoma, nodal preservation was noted in the first case whereas complete destruction of architecture was observed in the other [95]. The second case presented with lymphadenopathy and hepatosplenomegaly and had infiltration of lymphoid cells in the intrasinusoidal area of the lymph node. Predominant involvement of T zones was observed in one case [96]. Hence there may be two different patterns of presentation with diffuse pleomorphic involvement mimicking classical αβ T-cell lymphoma or hepatosplenic involvement mimicking hepatosplenic gamma-delta lymphoma [97].

The neoplastic cells express CD2, CD3, CD43, CD45. They also exhibit positivity for TIA-1, granzyme B and displayed a gamma delta phenotype (deltaTCR1+, Vdelta1+, Vdelta2−, Vdelta3−, betaF1−).

6.5.3 Genetic abnormality

The genotypic analysis shows TCR gamma-chain gene rearrangement pattern. The neoplastic cells also show expression of the latent membrane protein-1 by immunohistochemistry and EBV-encoded small RNAs by in situ hybridization. EBV positivity was also observed in tumor recurrence as reported in one case report [98]. A complex cytogenetic abnormality is seen in few cases, but no specific cytogenetic abnormality exists for this variant.

6.5.4 Clinical presentation

Patients most commonly present with lymphadenopathy. Usually, there is a past history of immunosuppression. In one case report, nodal gamma delta T-cell lymphoma presented post renal transplant in one case and after cytomegalovirus (CMV) infection in another case. Bone marrow infiltration and hepatosplenomegaly have also been reported [95].

6.5.5 Treatment and prognosis

This subtype is very resistant to conventional chemotherapy and has a very poor prognosis. Patients presenting with this type of lymphoma died within a short time after diagnosis [95].

7. Conclusion

Even though WHO 2016 classification of lymphoid malignancies recognizes four entities of gamma delta lymphomas, few more subtypes have been reported in literature which remains unclassified. These clinically important lymphomas pose a clinical challenge in diagnosis and management due to rarity and critical gap in consensus of treatment. Combination of clinical picture, morphology, immunophenotyping, molecular techniques are used in combination due to the diagnostic difficulties of these lymphomas. The poor prognosis associated with these subtypes is related to the rapidly evolving clinical picture and refractoriness to standard chemotherapies. Cytarabine combined with platinum-based regimen followed by stem cell transplantation seems to be the optimal management option for eligible patients. Encouraging prompt reporting of these rarer entities needs to be encouraged to further advance our understanding thus allowing newer perspective in the management.

Acknowledgements

1. Ramachandran Lakshmipathy, FRCPath, Bristol, UK.

2. Saravanan S. Karuppagounder, PhD, Burke Neurological Institute and Brain and Mind Research Institute, Weill Cornell Medicine, White Plains, NY 10605.

3. Oleg Reznik, Illustrator.

Conflict of interest

None.

Author details

Preethi Ramachandran[1*], Alok Aggarwal[2] and Jen Chin Wang[1]

1 Division of Hematology/Oncology, Brookdale University Hospital Medical Center, Brooklyn, New York, USA

2 Department of Hepatobiliary and General Surgery, Brookdale University Hospital and Medical Center, Brooklyn, New York, USA

*Address all correspondence to: drpreethiram@hotmail.com

References

[1] Wang SS, Vose JM. Epidemiology and prognosis of T-cell lymphoma. In: Foss F, editor. T-Cell Lymphomas. Totowa, NJ: Humana Press; 2013. pp. 25-39

[2] Swerdlow SH, Campo E, Pileri SA, et al. The 2016 revision of the World Health Organization classification of lymphoid neoplasms. Blood. 2016;**127**:2375-2390

[3] Bordessoule D, Gaulard P, Mason DY. Preferential localisation of human lymphocytes bearing gamma delta T cell receptors to the red pulp of the spleen. Journal of Clinical Pathology. 1990;**43**(6):461-464

[4] Sindhu H, Chen R, Chen H, Wong J, Chaudhry R, Xu Y, et al. Gamma-delta (gammadelta) T-cell lymphoma— Another case unclassifiable by World Health Organization classification: A case report. Journal of Medical Case Reports. 2017;**11**(1):163

[5] Kindt TJ, Goldsby RA, Osborne BA, Kuby J. Kuby Immunology. USA: Macmillan; 2007. p. 223. ISBN 978-1-4292-0211-4 [Retrieved 28 November 2010]

[6] Janeway CA Jr, Travers P, Walport M, et al. Immunobiology: The Immune System in Health and Disease. 5th ed. USA: Glossary, Garland Science; 2001

[7] Kreslavsky T, Gleimer M, Garbe AI, von Boehmer H. Alphabeta versus gammadelta fate choice: Counting the T-cell lineages at the branch point. Immunological Reviews. 2010;**238**(1):169-181

[8] Bluestone JA, Khattri R, Sciammas R, Sperling AI. TCR gamma delta cells: A specialized T-cell subset in the immune system. Annual Review of Cell and Developmental Biology. 1995;**11**:307-353

[9] Holtmeier W, Kabelitz D. Gammadelta T cells link innate and adaptive immune responses. Chemical Immunology and Allergy. 2005;**86**:151-183

[10] Hoft DF, Brown RM, Roodman ST. Bacille Calmette-Guerin vaccination enhances human gamma delta T cell responsiveness to mycobacteria suggestive of a memory-like phenotype. Journal of Immunology. 1998;**161**(2):1045-1054

[11] Boismenu R, Havran WL. An innate view of gamma delta T cells. Current Opinion in Immunology. 1997;**9**(1):57-63

[12] Williams N. T cells on the mucosal frontline. Science. 1998;**280**(5361):198-200

[13] Born WK, Reardon CL, O'Brien RL. The function of gammadelta T cells in innate immunity. Current Opinion in Immunology. 2006;**18**(1):31-38

[14] Tripodo C, Iannitto E, Florena AM, Pucillo CE, Piccaluga PP, Franco V, et al. Gamma-delta T-cell lymphomas. Nature Reviews. Clinical Oncology. 2009;**6**(12):707-717

[15] Rajoriya N, Fergusson JR, Leithead JA, Klenerman P. Gamma Delta T-lymphocytes in hepatitis C and chronic liver disease. Frontiers in Immunology. 2014;**5**:400

[16] Toro JR, Liewehr DJ, Pabby N, Sorbara L, Raffeld M, Steinberg SM, et al. Gamma-delta T-cell phenotype is associated with significantly decreased survival in cutaneous T-cell lymphoma. Blood. 2003;**101**(9):3407-3412

[17] Sabattini E, Bacci F, Sagramoso C, Pileri SA. WHO classification of tumours of haematopoietic and lymphoid tissues in 2008: An overview. Pathologica. 2010;**102**(3):83-87

[18] Miyazaki K et al. Gene expression profiling of peripheral T-cell lymphoma including γδ T-cell lymphoma. Blood. 2009;**113**(5):1071-1074

[19] Ferreri AJ, Govi S, Pileri SA. Hepatosplenic gamma-delta T-cell lymphoma. Critical Reviews in Oncology/Hematology. 2012;**83**(2):283-292

[20] Belhadj K, Reyes F, Farcet JP, Tilly H, Bastard C, Angonin R, et al. Hepatosplenic gammadelta T-cell lymphoma is a rare clinicopathologic entity with poor outcome: Report on a series of 21 patients. Blood. 2003;**102**(13):4261-4269

[21] Gaulard P, Bourquelot P, Kanavaros P, Haioun C, Le Couedic JP, Divine M, et al. Expression of the alpha/beta and gamma/delta T-cell receptors in 57 cases of peripheral T-cell lymphomas. Identification of a subset of gamma/delta T-cell lymphomas. The American Journal of Pathology. 1990;**137**(3):617-628

[22] Weidmann E. Hepatosplenic T cell lymphoma. A review on 45 cases since the first report describing the disease as a distinct lymphoma entity in 1990. Leukemia. 2000;**14**(6):991-997

[23] Campo E, Swerdlow SH, Harris NL, Pileri S, Stein H, Jaffe ES. The 2008 WHO classification of lymphoid neoplasms and beyond: Evolving concepts and practical applications. Blood. 2011;**117**(19):5019-5032

[24] Mackey AC, Green L, Liang LC, Dinndorf P, Avigan M. Hepatosplenic T cell lymphoma associated with infliximab use in young patients treated for inflammatory bowel disease. Journal of Pediatric Gastroenterology and Nutrition. 2007;**44**(2):265-267

[25] Ozaki S, Ogasahara K, Kosaka M, Inoshita T, Wakatsuki S, Uehara H, et al. Hepatosplenic gamma delta T-cell lymphoma associated with hepatitis B virus infection. The Journal of Medical Investigation. 1998;**44**(3-4):215-217

[26] de Wolf-Peeters C, Achten R. Gammadelta T-cell lymphomas: A homogeneous entity? Histopathology. 2000;**36**(4):294-305

[27] Cooke CB, Krenacs L, Stetler-Stevenson M, Greiner TC, Raffeld M, Kingma DW, et al. Hepatosplenic T-cell lymphoma: A distinct clinicopathologic entity of cytotoxic gamma delta T-cell origin. Blood. 1996;**88**(11):4265-4274

[28] Farcet JP, Gaulard P, Marolleau JP, Le Couedic JP, Henni T, Gourdin MF, et al. Hepatosplenic T-cell lymphoma: Sinusal/sinusoidal localization of malignant cells expressing the T-cell receptor gamma delta. Blood. 1990;**75**(11):2213-2219

[29] Swerdlow S, McColl K, Rong Y, Lam M, Gupta A, Distelhorst CW. Apoptosis inhibition by Bcl-2 gives way to autophagy in glucocorticoid-treated lymphocytes. Autophagy. 2008;**4**(5):612-620

[30] Alonsozana EL, Stamberg J, Kumar D, Jaffe ES, Medeiros LJ, Frantz C, et al. Isochromosome 7q: The primary cytogenetic abnormality in hepatosplenic gammadelta T cell lymphoma. Leukemia. 1997;**11**(8):1367-1372

[31] Colwill R, Dube I, Scott JG, Bailey D, Deharven E, Carstairs K, et al. Isochromosome 7q as the sole abnormality in an unusual case of T-cell lineage malignancy. Hematologic Pathology. 1990;**4**(1):53-58

[32] Jonveaux P, Daniel MT, Martel V, Maarek O, Berger R. Isochromosome 7q and trisomy 8 are consistent primary, non-random chromosomal abnormalities associated with hepatosplenic T gamma/delta lymphoma. Leukemia. 1996;**10**(9):1453-1455

[33] Finalet Ferreiro J, Rouhigharabaei L, Urbankova H, et al. Integrative Genomic and Transcriptomic Analysis Identified Candidate Genes Implicated in the Pathogenesis of Hepatosplenic T-Cell Lymphoma. Hoheisel JD, ed. PLoS ONE. 2014;**9**(7):e102977. DOI: 10.1371/journal.pone.0102977

[34] McKinney M, Moffitt AB, Gaulard P, et al. The genetic basis of hepatosplenic T cell lymphoma. Cancer Discovery. 2017;7(4):369-379. DOI: 10.1158/2159-8290.CD-16-0330

[35] Khong PL, Pang CB, Liang R, Kwong YL, Au WY. Fluorine-18 fluorodeoxyglucose positron emission tomography in mature T-cell and natural killer cell malignancies. Annals of Hematology. 2008;**87**:613-621

[36] Kako S, Izutsu K, Ota Y, Minatani Y, Sugaya M, Momose T, et al. FDG-PET in T-cell and NK-cell neoplasms. Annals of Oncology. 2007;**18**(10):1685-1690

[37] Storto G, Di Giorgio E, De Renzo A, Pizzuti LM, Cerciello G, Nardelli A, et al. Assessment of metabolic activity by PET-CT with F-18-FDG in patients with T-cell lymphoma. British Journal of Haematology. 2010;**151**(2):195-197

[38] Carbone PP, Kaplan HS, Musshoff K, Smithers DW, Tubiana M. Report of the committee on Hodgkin's disease staging classification. Cancer Research. 1971;**31**(11):1860-1861

[39] Gaulard P, de Leval L. Pathology of peripheral T-cell lymphomas: Where do we stand? Seminars in Hematology. 2014;**51**:5-16

[40] Kanavaros P, Farcet JP, Gaulard P, Haioun C, Divine M, Le Couedic JP, et al. Recombinative events of the T cell antigen receptor delta gene in peripheral T cell lymphomas. The Journal of Clinical Investigation. 1991;**87**(2):666-672

[41] Przybylski GK, Wu H, Macon WR, Finan J, Leonard DG, Felgar RE, et al. Hepatosplenic and subcutaneous panniculitis-like gamma/delta T cell lymphomas are derived from different Vdelta subsets of gamma/delta T lymphocytes. The Journal of Molecular Diagnostics. 2000;**2**(1):11-19

[42] Gaulard P, Belhadj K, Reyes F. Gammadelta T-cell lymphomas. Seminars in Hematology. 2003;**40**(3):233-243

[43] Sallah S, Smith SV, Lony LC, Woodard P, Schmitz JL, Folds JD. Gamma/delta T-cell hepatosplenic lymphoma: Review of the literature, diagnosis by flow cytometry and concomitant autoimmune hemolytic anemia. Annals of Hematology. 1997;**74**(3):139-142

[44] Vega F, Medeiros LJ, Bueso-Ramos C, Jones D, Lai R, Luthra R, et al. Hepatosplenic gamma/delta T-cell lymphoma in bone marrow. A sinusoidal neoplasm with blastic cytologic features. American Journal of Clinical Pathology. 2001;**116**(3):410-419

[45] Florena AM, Tripodo C, Porcasi R, Ingrao S, Fadda MR, De Cantis S, et al. Immunophenotypic profile and role of adhesion molecules in splenic marginal zone lymphoma with bone marrow involvement. Leukemia & Lymphoma. 2006;**47**(1):49-57

[46] Petit B, Leroy K, Kanavaros P, Boulland ML, Druet-Cabanac M, Haioun C, et al. Expression of p53 protein in T- and natural killer-cell lymphomas is associated with some clinicopathologic entities but rarely related to p53 mutations. Human Pathology. 2001;**32**(2):196-204

[47] Sayers TJ, Brooks AD, Ward JM, Hoshino T, Bere WE, Wiegand GW, et al. The restricted expression of granzyme M in human lymphocytes. Journal of Immunology. 2001;**166**(2):765-771

[48] Mittal S, Milner BJ, Johnston PW, Culligan DJ. A case of hepatosplenic

gamma-delta T-cell lymphoma with a transient response to fludarabine and alemtuzumab. European Journal of Haematology. 2006;**76**(6):531-534

[49] Jaeger G, Bauer F, Brezinschek R, Beham-Schmid C, Mannhalter C, Neumeister P. Hepatosplenic gammadelta T-cell lymphoma successfully treated with a combination of alemtuzumab and cladribine. Annals of Oncology. 2008;**19**(5):1025-1026

[50] Chanan-Khan A, Islam T, Alam A, Miller KC, Gibbs J, Barcos M, et al. Long-term survival with allogeneic stem cell transplant and donor lymphocyte infusion following salvage therapy with anti-CD52 monoclonal antibody (Campath) in a patient with alpha/beta hepatosplenic T-cell non-Hodgkin's lymphoma. Leukemia & Lymphoma. 2004;**45**(8):1673-1675

[51] Ooi J, Iseki T, Adachi D, Yamashita T, Tomonari A, Tojo A, et al. Successful allogeneic bone marrow transplantation for hepatosplenic gammadelta T cell lymphoma. Haematologica. 2001;**86**(10):E25

[52] Voss MH, Lunning MA, Maragulia JC, Papadopoulos EB, Goldberg J, Zelenetz AD, et al. Intensive induction chemotherapy followed by early high-dose therapy and hematopoietic stem cell transplantation results in improved outcome for patients with hepatosplenic T-cell lymphoma: A single institution experience. Clinical Lymphoma, Myeloma & Leukemia. 2013;**13**(1):8-14

[53] Advani RH, Hong F, Horning SJ, Kahl BS, Manola J, Swinnen LJ, et al. Cardiac toxicity associated with bevacizumab (Avastin) in combination with CHOP chemotherapy for peripheral T cell lymphoma in ECOG 2404 trial. Leukemia & Lymphoma. 2012;**53**(4):718-720

[54] Zinzani PL, Musuraca G, Tani M, Stefoni V, Marchi E, Fina M, et al. Phase II trial of proteasome inhibitor bortezomib in patients with relapsed or refractory cutaneous T-cell lymphoma. Journal of Clinical Oncology. 2007;**25**(27):4293-4297

[55] Dueck G, Chua N, Prasad A, Finch D, Stewart D, White D, et al. Interim report of a phase 2 clinical trial of lenalidomide for T-cell non-Hodgkin lymphoma. Cancer. 2010;**116**(19):4541-4548

[56] Zinzani PL, Pellegrini C, Broccoli A, Stefoni V, Gandolfi L, Quirini F, et al. Lenalidomide monotherapy for relapsed/refractory peripheral T-cell lymphoma not otherwise specified. Leukemia & Lymphoma. 2011;**52**(8):1585-1588

[57] O'Connor OA, Pro B, Pinter-Brown L, Bartlett N, Popplewell L, Coiffier B, et al. Pralatrexate in patients with relapsed or refractory peripheral T-cell lymphoma: Results from the pivotal PROPEL study. Journal of Clinical Oncology. 2011;**29**(9):1182-1189

[58] Mann BS, Johnson JR, Cohen MH, Justice R, Pazdur R. FDA approval summary: Vorinostat for treatment of advanced primary cutaneous T-cell lymphoma. The Oncologist. 2007;**12**(10):1247-1252

[59] Woo S, Gardner ER, Chen X, Ockers SB, Baum CE, Sissung TM, et al. Population pharmacokinetics of romidepsin in patients with cutaneous T-cell lymphoma and relapsed peripheral T-cell lymphoma. Clinical Cancer Research. 2009;**15**(4):1496-1503

[60] Endly DC, Weenig RH, Peters MS, Viswanatha DS, Comfere NI. Indolent course of cutaneous gamma-delta T-cell lymphoma. Journal of Cutaneous Pathology. 2013;**40**(10):896-902

[61] Toro JR, Beaty M, Sorbara L, Turner ML, White J, Kingma DW, et al. Gamma delta T-cell lymphoma of the skin: A

clinical, microscopic, and molecular study. Archives of Dermatology. 2000;**136**(8):1024-1032

[62] Ralfkiaer E, Wollf-Sneedorff A, Thomsen K, Geisler C, Vejlsgaard GL. T-cell receptor gamma delta-positive peripheral T-cell lymphomas presenting in the skin: A clinical, histological and immunophenotypic study. Experimental Dermatology. 1992;**1**(1):31-36

[63] Yamamoto K, Matsuoka H, Yakushijin K, Funakoshi Y, Okamura A, Hayashi Y, et al. A novel five-way translocation, t(3;9;13;8;14)(q27;p13;q32;q24;q32), with concurrent MYC and BCL6 rearrangements in a primary bone marrow B-cell lymphoma. Cancer Genetics. 2011;**204**(9):501-506

[64] Kim YH, Willemze R, Pimpinelli N, Whittaker S, Olsen EA, Ranki A, et al. TNM classification system for primary cutaneous lymphomas other than mycosis fungoides and Sezary syndrome: A proposal of the International Society for Cutaneous Lymphomas (ISCL) and the cutaneous lymphoma task force of the European Organization of Research and Treatment of Cancer (EORTC). Blood. 2007;**110**(2):479-484

[65] Hoefnagel JJ, Vermeer MH, Jansen PM, Heule F, van Voorst Vader PC, Sanders CJ, et al. Primary cutaneous marginal zone B-cell lymphoma: Clinical and therapeutic features in 50 cases. Archives of Dermatology. 2005;**141**(9):1139-1145

[66] Arnulf B, Copie-Bergman C, Delfau-Larue MH, Lavergne-Slove A, Bosq J, Wechsler J, et al. Nonhepatosplenic gammadelta T-cell lymphoma: A subset of cytotoxic lymphomas with mucosal or skin localization. Blood. 1998;**91**(5):1723-1731

[67] Katoh A, Ohshima K, Kanda M, Haraoka S, Sugihara M, Suzumiya J, et al. Gastrointestinal T cell lymphoma: Predominant cytotoxic phenotypes, including alpha/beta, gamma/delta T cell and natural killer cells. Leukemia & Lymphoma. 2000;**39**(1-2):97-111

[68] Al Omran S, Mourad WA, Ali MA. Gamma/delta peripheral T-cell lymphoma of the breast diagnosed by fine-needle aspiration biopsy. Diagnostic Cytopathology. 2002;**26**(3):170-173

[69] Scolnik MP, Burgos RA, Paz A, Weinreiter M, del Carmen Ardaiz M, Bare P, et al. Nonhepatosplenic gamma delta T-cell lymphoma with initial testicular compromise. American Journal of Hematology. 2000;**65**(3):260-262

[70] Tsujikawa T, Itoh A, Bamba M, Andoh A, Hodohara K, Inoue H, et al. Aggressive jejunal gamma deltaT-cell lymphoma derived from intraepithelial lymphocytes: An autopsy case report. Journal of Gastroenterology. 1998;**33**(2):280-284

[71] Kumar S, Krenacs L, Medeiros J, Elenitoba-Johnson KS, Greiner TC, Sorbara L, et al. Subcutaneous panniculitic T-cell lymphoma is a tumor of cytotoxic T lymphocytes. Human Pathology. 1998;**29**(4):397-403

[72] Willemze R, Jansen PM, Cerroni L, Berti E, Santucci M, Assaf C, et al. Subcutaneous panniculitis-like T-cell lymphoma: Definition, classification, and prognostic factors: An EORTC cutaneous lymphoma group study of 83 cases. Blood. 2008;**111**(2):838-845

[73] Berti E, Cerri A, Cavicchini S, Delia D, Soligo D, Alessi E, et al. Primary cutaneous gamma/delta T-cell lymphoma presenting as disseminated pagetoid reticulosis. The Journal of Investigative Dermatology. 1991;**96**(5):718-723

[74] Go RS, Wester SM. Immunophenotypic and molecular

features, clinical outcomes, treatments, and prognostic factors associated with subcutaneous panniculitis-like T-cell lymphoma: A systematic analysis of 156 patients reported in the literature. Cancer. 2004;**101**(6):1404-1413

[75] Fujii M, Uehara J, Honma M, Ito Y, Takahashi H, Ishida-Yamamoto A, et al. Primary cutaneous gammadelta-T-cell lymphoma treated with low-dose methotrexate and narrowband ultraviolet B irradiation: Report of a case with testicular involvement. The Journal of Dermatology. 2011;**38**(4):368-372

[76] Mehta N, Wayne AS, Kim YH, Hale GA, Alvarado CS, Myskowski P, et al. Bexarotene is active against subcutaneous panniculitis-like T-cell lymphoma in adult and pediatric populations. Clinical Lymphoma, Myeloma & Leukemia. 2012;**12**(1):20-25

[77] Guitart J, Weisenburger DD, Subtil A, Kim E, Wood G, Duvic M, et al. Cutaneous gammadelta T-cell lymphomas: A spectrum of presentations with overlap with other cytotoxic lymphomas. The American Journal of Surgical Pathology. 2012;**36**(11):1656-1665

[78] Takeshita M, Imayama S, Oshiro Y, Kurihara K, Okamoto S, Matsuki Y, et al. Clinicopathologic analysis of 22 cases of subcutaneous panniculitis-like CD56− or CD56+ lymphoma and review of 44 other reported cases. American Journal of Clinical Pathology. 2004;**121**(3):408-416

[79] Ott MM, Ott G, Klinker H, Trunk MJ, Katzenberger T, Muller-Hermelink HK. Abdominal T-cell non-Hodgkin's lymphoma of the gamma/delta type in a patient with selective immunoglobulin A deficiency. The American Journal of Surgical Pathology. 1998;**22**(4):500-506

[80] Sandberg Y, Almeida J, Gonzalez M, Lima M, Barcena P, Szczepanski T, et al. TCRgammadelta+ large granular lymphocyte leukemias reflect the spectrum of normal antigen-selected TCRgammadelta+ T-cells. Leukemia. 2006;**20**(3):505-513

[81] Bourgault-Rouxel AS, Loughran TP Jr, Zambello R, Epling-Burnette PK, Semenzato G, Donadieu J, et al. Clinical spectrum of gammadelta+ T cell LGL leukemia: Analysis of 20 cases. Leukemia Research. 2008;**32**(1):45-48

[82] Makishima H, Ishida F, Saito H, Ichikawa N, Ozaki Y, Ito S, et al. Lymphoproliferative disease of granular lymphocytes with T-cell receptor gamma delta-positive phenotype: Restricted usage of T-cell receptor gamma and delta subunit genes. European Journal of Haematology. 2003;**70**(4):212-218

[83] Chen YH, Chadburn A, Evens AM, Winter JN, Gordon LI, Chenn A, et al. Clinical, morphologic, immunophenotypic, and molecular cytogenetic assessment of CD4-/CD8-gammadelta T-cell large granular lymphocytic leukemia. American Journal of Clinical Pathology. 2011;**136**(2):289-299

[84] Osuji N, Matutes E, Catovsky D, Lampert I, Wotherspoon A. Histopathology of the spleen in T-cell large granular lymphocyte leukemia and T-cell prolymphocytic leukemia: A comparative review. The American Journal of Surgical Pathology. 2005;**29**(7):935-941

[85] Gentile TC, Uner AH, Hutchison RE, Wright J, Ben-Ezra J, Russell EC, et al. CD3+, CD56+ aggressive variant of large granular lymphocyte leukemia. Blood. 1994;**84**(7):2315-2321

[86] Vartholomatos G, Alymara V, Dova L, Kolaitis N, Bourantas KL. T-cell receptor gammadelta-large granular lymphocytic leukemia associated with an aberrant phenotype and TCR-Vbeta20 clonality. Haematologica. 2004;**89**(5):ECR16

[87] Dhodapkar MV, Li CY, Lust JA, Tefferi A, Phyliky RL. Clinical spectrum of clonal proliferations of T-large granular lymphocytes: A T-cell clonopathy of undetermined significance? Blood. 1994;**84**(5):1620-1627

[88] Shichishima T, Kawaguchi M, Ono N, Oshimi K, Nakamura N, Maruyama Y. Gammadelta T-cell large granular lymphocyte (LGL) leukemia with spontaneous remission. American Journal of Hematology. 2004;**75**(3):168-172

[89] Takeuchi M, Tamaoki A, Soda R, Takahashi K. Spontaneous remission of large granular lymphocyte T cell leukemia. Leukemia. 1999;**13**(2):313-314

[90] Lamy T, Loughran TP Jr. Clinical features of large granular lymphocyte leukemia. Seminars in Hematology. 2003;**40**(3):185-195

[91] Osuji N, Matutes E, Tjonnfjord G, Grech H, Del Giudice I, Wotherspoon A, et al. T-cell large granular lymphocyte leukemia: A report on the treatment of 29 patients and a review of the literature. Cancer. 2006;**107**(3):570-578

[92] Gentile TC, Loughran TP Jr. Resolution of autoimmune hemolytic anemia following splenectomy in CD3+ large granular lymphocyte leukemia. Leukemia & Lymphoma. 1996;**23**(3-4):405-408

[93] Pandolfi F, Loughran TP Jr, Starkebaum G, Chisesi T, Barbui T, Chan WC, et al. Clinical course and prognosis of the lymphoproliferative disease of granular lymphocytes. A multicenter study. Cancer. 1990;**65**(2):341-348

[94] Alekshun TJ, Tao J, Sokol L. Aggressive T-cell large granular lymphocyte leukemia: A case report and review of the literature. American Journal of Hematology. 2007;**82**(6):481-485

[95] Charton-Bain MC, Brousset P, Bouabdallah R, Gaulard P, Merlio JP, Dubus P, et al. Variation in the histological pattern of nodal involvement by gamma/delta T-cell lymphoma. Histopathology. 2000;**36**(3):233-239

[96] Ohno T, Komada F, Yamaguchi M, Oka K, Nishii K, Tsuda M, et al. Gamma/delta T-cell lymphoma with hepatosplenomegaly: Report of a case. International Journal of Hematology. 1993;**57**(3):269-276

[97] Saito T, Matsuno Y, Tanosaki R, Watanabe T, Kobayashi Y, Tobinai K. Gamma delta T-cell neoplasms: A clinicopathological study of 11 cases. Annals of Oncology. 2002;**13**(11):1792-1798

[98] Kagami Y, Nakamura S, Suzuki R, Yatabe Y, Okada Y, Kobayasi T, et al. A nodal gamma/delta T-cell lymphoma with an association of Epstein-Barr virus. The American Journal of Surgical Pathology. 1997;**21**(6):729-736

Chapter 6

Precision Medicine Concepts in T-Cell Lymphoma

Philipp Staber

Abstract

Modern oncology witnesses an increasing number of new effective anticancer drugs targeting specific oncogenic pathways. Despite these advances, real-world experience with targeted single agents is disappointing since drug resistance usually occurs after a short time. This is particularly true for patients with refractory or relapsed T-cell lymphoma (TCL) who so far could not benefit from novel agents and demonstrate a short survival time of only 3 months. The novel genetic information gained from genome-wide high-throughput techniques has greatly improved our understanding of TCL. However, if precision medicine strategies are based solely on genetics, it runs into two major challenges: (1) the heterogeneity within the cancer of an individual patient and (2) the incomplete understanding of the degree of contribution of a specific mutation to a tumor phenotype. Next-generation functional drug screening (ngFDS) aims to address these problems. Studies that proof the clinical utility of ngFDS are currently limited. The following chapter aims to discuss recent advances of ngFDS and to line out its potential for TCL patients.

Keywords: T-cell lymphoma, precision medicine, genomics, transcriptomics, next-generation functional screening

1. Introduction

TCL is a heterogeneous group of rare lymphoid malignancies generally with dismal outcome [1, 2]. With current treatment options, a majority of patients do not achieve remission or experience relapse after completion of therapy [3–6]. Patients with newly diagnosed TCL are most commonly treated with anthracycline-based (CHOP-like) chemotherapy regimens, often followed by consolidation with high-dose chemotherapy and stem cell transplantation in eligible patients [1]. Patients with relapsed TCL have a dismal prognosis with a median overall survival of only 3 months [2]. Unfortunately, mechanisms of drug resistance in TCL leading to progression and relapse remain elusive, and predictive biomarkers do not exist, precluding clinical progress. Three major limitations have thus far hampered a systematic and causative understanding of drug resistance in TCL: (I) adherence to genetic studies and barriers in translating this genomic information into direct clinical benefit for patients, (II) as for functional analysis, a general adherence to cell lines that is prone to clonal artifacts and that not faithfully recapitulates relevant physiology, and (III) lack of considerable biobanks of viably frozen cells from fresh dissociated lymphomas. All three points are discussed in detail below.

2. Precision medicine concepts

2.1 Advances and shortcomings of genetic studies

Predicting clinical treatment outcome from detailed characterization of patient material is one of the key challenges of modern oncology. The most so-called precision medicine approaches either rely on correlation of clinical outcome with molecular profiles such as genetic mutations [7] or attempt to reproduce the disease in an ex vivo model system and extrapolate from measured drug response to the patient outcome [8, 9]. Genetic approaches are state of the art for most diseases and have also been successful in some indications (e.g., targeting BCR-ABL with imatinib in chronic myeloid leukemia (CML)). TCLs, however, as most cancers, categorically differ from the rare monogenetic disease model and are driven by microevolutionary processes leading to broad genetic heterogeneity [10] and making a purely correlational logic extremely challenging [11].

Recent sequencing studies in TCL confirmed a set of genetic alterations in specific subtypes, including recurrent mutations in the epigenetic modifiers TET2, IDH2, and DNMT3A and the small GTPase RhoA in angioimmunoblastic T-cell lymphoma (AITL) [12–15], while JAK/STAT pathway alterations through mutations at various levels seem to be present across all TCL subtypes, particularly in anaplastic large cell lymphoma (ALCL) [16]. For the most common subtypes of TCL, including peripheral T-cell lymphoma not otherwise specified (PTCL-NOS), AITL, and ALCL, genetic data are largely based on targeted DNA sequencing approaches focusing on mutations in pre-selected panels of genes, while unbiased sequencing approaches like whole exome sequencing are only available in small cohorts. Previous studies in ALK-ALCL utilizing immunohistochemistry and fluorescence in situ hybridization identified for ~38% of the patients with ALK- ALCL DUSP22- and TP63-rearrangements to be associated with good prognosis as for DUSP22- or with exceptional dismal prognosis as for TP63- rearrangements when receiving CHOP-like regimens [17].

Despite the significant amount of recurrent mutations in genes involved in DNA methylation like DNMT3A, TET2, or IDH2, no genome-wide epigenetic profiling has been reported in a sufficient amount of clinically well-annotated samples [12, 13, 18]. Therefore, we currently only can assume that broad epigenetic changes are frequent in TCL. In contrast to B-cell lymphoma, relatively strong responses to epigenetic modifying agents, such as HDAC inhibitors and methylation modifiers, are clinically evident [19–21].

Thus, there is evidence that in TCL the epigenome is of particular importance; however, systematic studies on epigenetic profiling in TCL are lacking and so are direct connections of genetic mutations in epigenetic modifiers and clinical responses to epigenetic drugs. A comprehensive characterization of genetic and epigenetic alterations and clinical response to specific drugs is highly warranted for TCL.

2.2 Advances and shortcomings of functional studies

Despite significant success to identify genomic alterations that might establish and drive hematologic malignancies, genetic studies face problems in translating genomic information into drug-able targets to directly benefit the patients. Results of personal medical efforts in cancer patients so far are sometimes promising but with the majority rather appearing disappointing [22–26]. In a landmark study that used each patient as their own control, Von Hoff et al. reported that 27% of patients with recurrent metastatic cancer of any kind had a 30% longer progression-free survival (PFS) with treatment selected on the basis of genetic profiling than they did with their previous treatment [25].

The first randomized trial of genomic-based precision medicine, the SHIVA study, did not use patients as their own control but investigated the effect of genetic marker-based targeted treatment comparing with treatment at physician's choice in heavily pretreated patients with cancer. The SHIVA study failed to demonstrate a benefit for patients treated with genetic precision treatment [26]. We need to consider that our knowledge of how cancer genotype relates to its phenotype and of the complexity of the dynamic microevolutionary procedures that occur in an individual cancer is very limited [10].

Therefore, dynamic approaches that measure drug responses in cancer cells derived from patient biopsies promise to complement the static molecular measurements. Functional approaches could contribute important information to improve the selection of the right drug for the right patient at the right time. For instance, ex vivo chemosensitivity tests have been performed in samples of patients suffering chronic or acute leukemia [8, 27–30] and also in gut stem cell-derived organoids [31, 32], in breast cancer cell lines [33], and in xenografted mice [34, 35]. All these pioneering functional studies have not been integrated into clinical routine, but they provided proof of concept for ex vivo responses that may match clinical response. However, due to the extensive time of the assays used, the clinical benefits were limited [36–38]. First proof of concept data was obtained with functional screens detecting drug activity in cell cultures with luminescent assays that predicted activity and resistance to drugs in patients [9] and leading to initiation of a clinical trial for targeted therapy of relapsed acute myeloid leukemia [39].

In two recent reports, luminescent assay-based drug profiling has also been performed in a T-cell neoplasm and in T-cell prolymphocytic leukemia (T-PLL) [40, 41]. T-PLL is a rare, clinically heterogenous neoplasm, which is treated with alemtuzumab-based induction in patients with symptoms, followed by consolidative stem cell transplantation [42]. There are no randomized controlled trials that inform the management of T-PLL; thus it is an area of clear unmet need. Boidol et al. used single-cell suspensions from fresh bone marrow, peripheral blood, or lymph node samples from 86 patients and exposed cells to 106 different compounds to perform functional drug screening after 72 hours [41]. Cancer cell-specific responses were calculated from individual dose-response curves, and tissue microarrays were generated for comparative protein expression profiling (**Figure 1**).

BCL-2 inhibitor venetoclax exhibited the strongest differential response for T-PLL (**Figure 2**). Ex vivo responses to venetoclax significantly correlated with BCL-2 protein expression scores but not with scores for BCL-2 gene family members BCL-XL and MCL-1. BCL-XL and MCL-1 expression scores demonstrated a significant correlation, while only MCL-1 appears to be inversely correlated with BCL-2 expression. T-PLL samples were among the entities with the highest BCL-2 scores, showing the most dramatic response to BCL-2 inhibition via venetoclax. Importantly, the second ex vivo dug screening report on T-PLL also found consistent activities of BCL-2 inhibition in T-PLL, thus confirming these results in an independent cohort [40] (**Figure 2**). It also demonstrates the reliability and reproducibility of functional assays.

It is noteworthy that luminescent assay-based functional assays can recapitulate differential responses to venetoclax of specific disease entities experienced in the clinic. High-resolution dose-response curves of venetoclax clearly distinguished CLL, AML, and T-PLL samples (**Figure 3**). As expected from clinical data, CLL samples demonstrated pronounced effects at already very discrete doses (50% inhibitory concentration [IC50], around 5 nM). In contrast AML samples responded at high concentrations (median IC50: 10 μM). Response curves of T-PLL samples were in the middle of AML and CLL samples (median IC50: 1 μM).

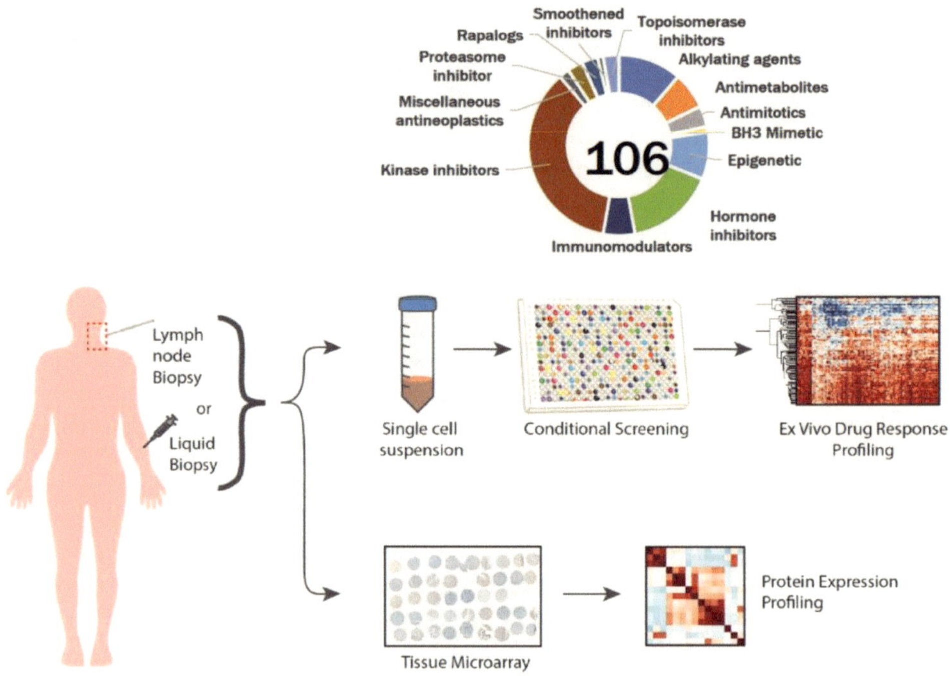

Figure 1.
Workflow: After sampling, single cell suspensions are used for high-throughput drug-screening. Formaldehyde conserved samples are processed for tissue microarrays for comparative protein expression profiling.

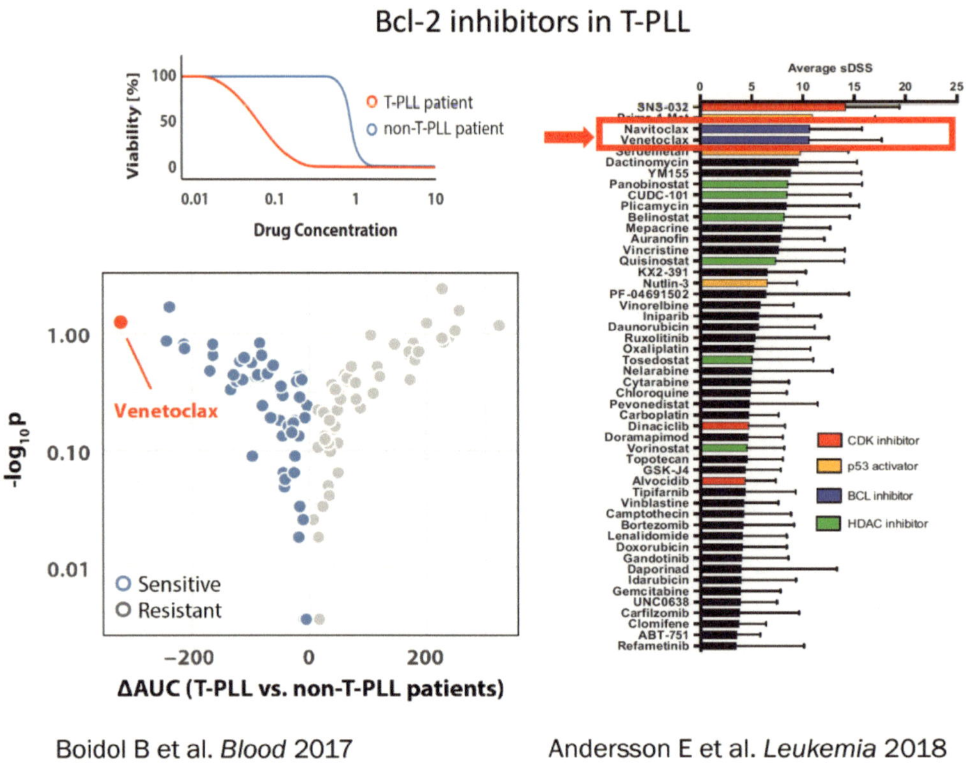

Figure 2.
Cancer cell-specific responses were calculated from individual dose-response curves in two independent publications. In both, drug-profiling revealed that BCL-2 inhibitor venetoclax exhibited a significant differential response for T-PLL.

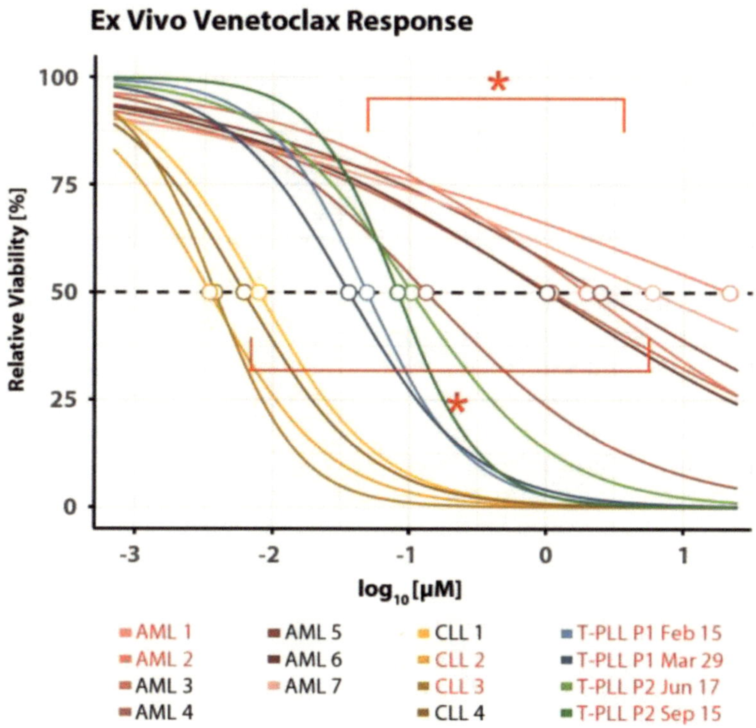

Figure 3.
High-resolution dose-response curves of venetoclax in CLL, AML, and T-PLL samples.

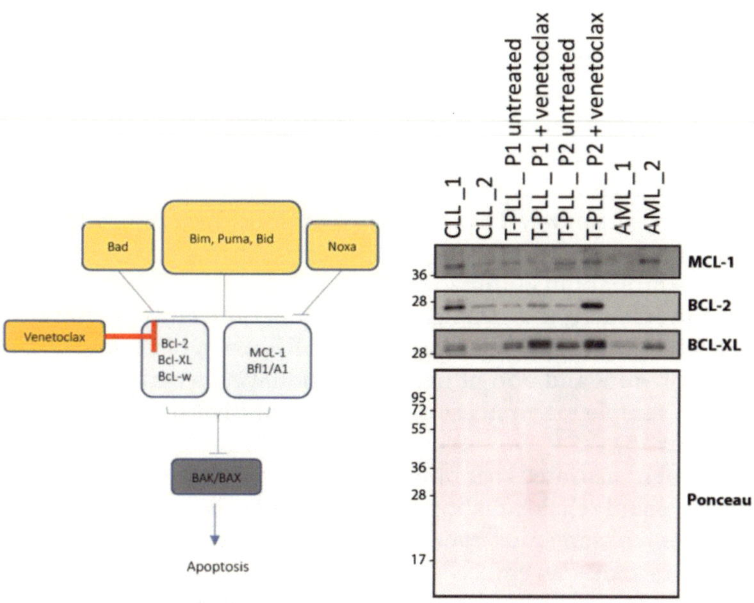

Figure 4.
Venetoclax treatment induced BCL-2 and BCL-XL protein expression.

Trying to elucidate the mechanisms, we investigated the protein expression of other BCL-2 family members. Interestingly venetoclax treatment induced BCL-2 and BCL-XL protein expression in the two patients, since MCL-1 levels did not changed. Therefore BCL-XL upregulation could be a potential mechanism of venetoclax resistance, and the additional use of drugs targeting BCL-XL or suppressing BCL-XL could be mechanistically synergistic (**Figure 4**).

Therefore, studies testing venetoclax with appropriate combination partners in T-PLL are warranted. Combination therapies are essential to overcome the resistance mechanisms that limit the long-term efficacy of conventional cytotoxic chemotherapies or targeted agents inhibiting single pathways. It is important to establish a workflow to systematically test multiple drug combinations and applied it to successfully identify synergistic combinations [43]. The main challenges to systematic large-scale drug-drug combination testing are that the number of two-drug combination remains in tens of thousands, thus limiting the numbers of combinations to be tested in primary patient material. To overcome this burden, the community continues to develop innovative computational approaches for preselecting sets of putative synergistic drugs involving network analysis, dynamic modeling, and high-content machine learning. However, based mainly on genetic data, only approx. 40% in silico predicted drug synergies are confirmed by ex vivo combination testing as demonstrated at the example of T-cell prolymphocytic leukemia (T-PLL) [44]. A reason for the rather low functional confirmation rate could be the low correlation between high-throughput ex vivo drug testing and mutation profiling [40]. It is therefore tempting to propose a smart way to preselect combination partners that are then analyzed in vitro.

2.3 Advances of single-cell functional studies

Luminescent assay-based functional assays have the big plus of high-throughput because full automation is more easily established. However, these assays cannot provide data at the single-cell level and thus no data on individual cell based functional information. Especially if the aim is to address the heterogeneity within one individual patient, i.e., to discriminate malignant and normal cells or to use complex co-culture systems, investigators could be interested in automated microscopic imaging technology. Minimally invasive protocols could provide drug-response information in co-culture systems. This could maintain leukemia and multiple myeloma cells for a longer cultivating time and enhance the screening capabilities of patient samples [45–47]. Snijder and colleagues investigated the clinical impact of a newly developed single-cell image analysis technology platform that operates using a combination of multi-parametric immunofluorescence and high-throughput automated microscopy [48]. In contrast to functional methods used previously, this next-generation functional drug screening (ngFDS) technique allows a fast tumor cell -specific quantification of biological parameters of millions of adherent and non-adherent individual cells with high sample efficiency, minimal sample manipulation, extensive automation, and fast turnaround times [49] (**Figure 5**).

The authors demonstrated that multi-parametric, image-based, immunophenotypic cytometry could reliably distinguish malignant cells from normal bystander cells in a high-content screening context. They showed how this approach can detect phenotypes across several cellular compartments, quantifying, for example, T-cell engagement by the bispecific, CD19-directed, T-cell engager blinatumomab in patient samples. They applied the method to patients with aggressive hematologic malignancies failing at least two lines of therapy and without further standard treatment options. These patients will usually receive either best available therapy or best supportive care or will be enrolled in clinical trials. Upon relapse, blood, bone marrow, pleural effusions, or excised lymph node biopsies were collected depending on the disease manifestation. The primary endpoints were to evaluate the feasibility of integrating ngFDS into the clinic and to assess clinical response in patients who received a treatment according to ngFDS results as an individual healing attempt [49] (**Figure 6**).

This prospective single-center pilot study demonstrates that it is possible to integrate automated microscopy-based next-generation functional drug screening (ngFDS) for patients with aggressive hematologic malignancies into the clinical routine. Importantly, the ngFDS results suggested treatment regimens that lead to an improved ORR and longer PFS for patients than the last treatment regimen the patients had just experienced progression on (**Figure 7**). These results demonstrate that we are already in possession of a wide array of working chemotherapeutics and

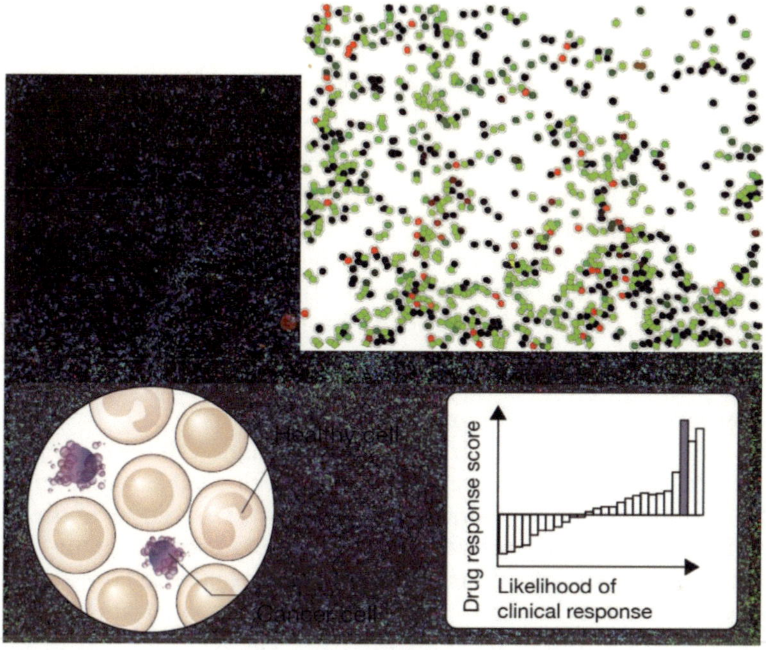

Figure 5.
Next-generation functional drug screening (ngFDS) technique allows a fast tumor cell-specific quantification of biological parameters of millions of adherent and non-adherent individual cells.

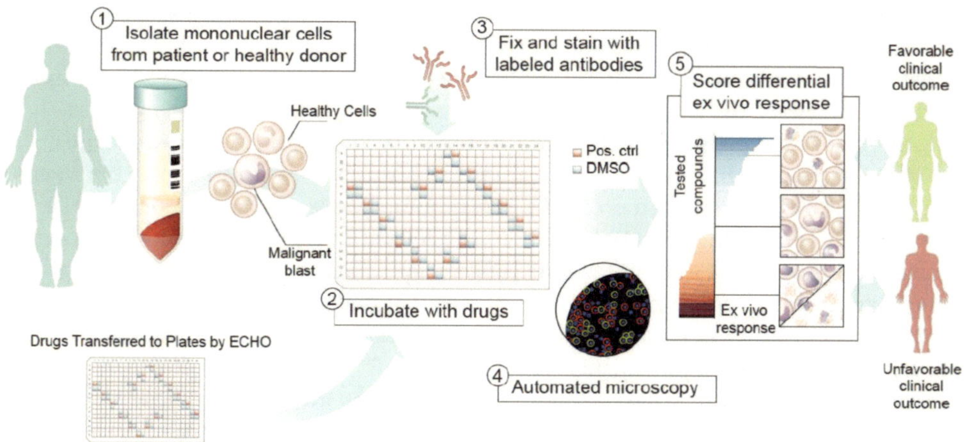

Figure 6.
Blood, bone marrow, pleural effusions, or excised lymph node biopsies were collected depending on the disease manifestation. The primary endpoints were to evaluate the feasibility of integrating ngFDS into the clinic and to assess clinical response.

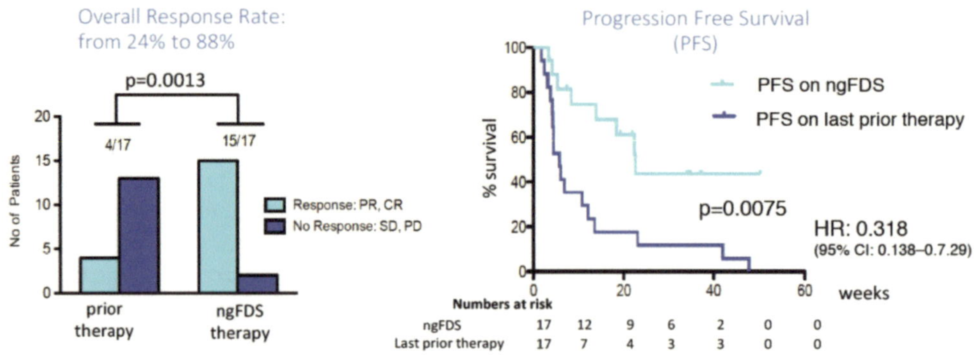

Figure 7.
ngFDS results suggested treatment regimens that lead to an improved ORR and longer PFS for patients than the last treatment regimen the patients had just experienced progression on.

targeted inhibitors that in principle are capable of breaking drug resistance even in multi-refractory cancers, given that we identify the right drugs for each individual patient, at the right time during their treatment.

The study name is EXALT for extended analysis for leukemia/lymphoma treatment. It is a prospective non-randomized study with each patient functioning as their own control, thus allowing to determine the overall effect across heterogeneous disease entities and different therapies. The nonexistence of randomization could harbor a bias. In future studies testing ngFDS-guided therapies, randomization and physician choice are warranted.

Image-based quantification of drug effects with single-cell resolution in patient biopsies, as introduced here, represents a robust and clinically useful platform to assign powerful individualized therapeutic regimens. The strength of the approach resides in the statistical power derived from monitoring with computer-aided precision millions of individual functional events, i.e., single-cell drug responses, combined with the ability to discriminate cell types, allowing to score specific rather than general and averaged cytotoxic effects. The approach may be valuable for the personalized identification of clinically effective therapies for many other hematological malignancies, especially for rare diseases, like TCL. The selection of personalized therapy by ngFDS benefits from the ability to measure hundreds to thousands of drug exposures using small patient samples, where each ex vivo treatment includes healthy-cell-controls from the same patient sample. This allows for direct estimation of the therapeutic window, while the minimal ex vivo culturing of cells and compatibility with clinical diagnostic markers ensure fast and relevant feedback. Further, the platform can take advantage of the use of liquid biopsies where small target cells can be detected. These integrated drug response profiles, or "chemotypes," of individual people are the culmination of the interplay between a number of molecular parameters of the responding cells, including not only the genetic, proteomic, and metabolic state of the cells but also the direct and indirect molecular interactions with other cells [48], recapitulating relevant physiological complexity. Such chemotypes may offer functional insight into the underlying health status of an individual, with potentially wide-ranging implications also in preventative and participatory medicine.

As shown here, ngFDS can provide clinically useful guidance in the absence of genetic information. However, the full potential of the approach will certainly be realized only through the synergy with genomic and other molecular patient profiling. This could lead to highly accurate personalized treatments, coupled with companion diagnostics, as well as powerful route to mechanistic elucidation of gene-to-phenotype relationships.

2.4 Outlook for precision medicine in TCL

Collectively, the combination of advanced functional strategies, chemical genetics, and phenotypic screening approaches to holistically chart and chemically probe mechanisms of drug failure opens fundamental new treatment opportunities for TCL patients. Phenotypic single-cell drug screening is a highly innovative approach that helps to identify sensitive drugs and proved to be effective in late-stage hematological malignancies [49]. The next step to achieve the real treatment goal of a "long-term remission" is to identify a systematic way to identify mechanistically grounded effective drug-drug combinations. Clinically fully annotated viable sample sets consisting of sufficient TCL samples will provide the basis to probe with the help of network analysis, dynamic modeling, and high-content machine learning a useful algorithm for individual combination treatment to tackle drug resistance up-front.

Novelty emerges from the innovative intersection of cutting edge technologies, such as an innovative drug screening pipeline at cellular resolution, the use of novel immune competent xenograft mouse models that recapitulate human immune response, and single-cell RNAseq applied in primary TCL cells upon multiple drug perturbations. Foremost, it will be important to probe these data sets with cutting edge bioinformatics and network medicine pipelines.

ngFDS will give hemato-oncologists a new tool to identify the most promising treatment combinations to help overcome resistance in otherwise refractory TCLs on a patient-to-patient basis. The success of ngFDS, added a new layer to how doctors can base treatment decisions, since it significantly improved the patients' outcome [49]. A rational guidance to pick the most appropriate combination partner promises to achieve long-term remissions.

I further expect that the established pipelines of ex vivo testing identified drug combinations will outline and instruct prospective clinical trials as has recently shown [41, 45] (approval and funding of a clinical study starting Q4 2018: venetoclax + ibrutinib in T-PLL (VIT-study;) Ph2 Study M18–803 (AbbVie) = the first global clinical trial for T-PLL).

Finally, ngFDS challenges the concepts of future clinical trial design. It requires a study design that provides the highest possible flexibility for experimental treatment to allow data-guided combination of targeted agents with antibody-based therapies for TCL. Larger prospective studies should focus on specific disease entities and randomize between arms of different treatment selection procedures to capture the full potential of functional assays for our TCL patients.

Author details

Philipp Staber
Division of Hematology and Hemostaseology, Department of Medicine I, Medical University of Vienna, Vienna, Austria

*Address all correspondence to: philipp.staber@meduniwien.ac.at

References

[1] d'Amore F et al. Peripheral T-cell lymphomas: ESMO clinical practice guidelines for diagnosis, treatment and follow-up. Annals of Oncology. 2015;**26**(Suppl 5):v108-v115

[2] Mak V et al. Survival of patients with peripheral T-cell lymphoma after first relapse or progression: Spectrum of disease and rare long-term survivors. Journal of Clinical Oncology. 2013;**31**(16):1970-1976

[3] Swerdlow SH et al. The 2016 revision of the World Health Organization classification of lymphoid neoplasms. Blood. 2016;**127**(20):2375-2390

[4] de Leval L et al. Angioimmunoblastic T-cell lymphoma is the most common T-cell lymphoma in two distinct French information data sets. Haematologica. 2015;**100**(9):e361-e364

[5] Vose J et al. International peripheral T-cell and natural killer/T-cell lymphoma study: Pathology findings and clinical outcomes. Journal of Clinical Oncology. 2008;**26**(25):4124-4130

[6] Moskowitz AJ, Lunning MA, Horwitz SM. How I treat the peripheral T-cell lymphomas. Blood. 2014;**123**(17):2636-2644

[7] Schilsky RL. Personalized medicine in oncology: The future is now. Nature Reviews. Drug Discovery. 2010;**9**(5):363-366

[8] Montero J et al. Drug-induced death signaling strategy rapidly predicts cancer response to chemotherapy. Cell. 2015;**160**(5):977-989

[9] Pemovska T et al. Individualized systems medicine strategy to tailor treatments for patients with chemorefractory acute myeloid leukemia. Cancer Discovery. 2013; **3**(12):1416-1429

[10] Friedman AA et al. Precision medicine for cancer with next-generation functional diagnostics. Nature Reviews. Cancer. 2015;**15**(12): 747-756

[11] Urbach D et al. Cancer heterogeneity: Origins and implications for genetic association studies. Trends in Genetics. 2012;**28**(11):538-543

[12] Sakata-Yanagimoto M et al. Somatic RHOA mutation in angioimmunoblastic T cell lymphoma. Nature Genetics. 2014;**46**(2):171-175

[13] Palomero T et al. Recurrent mutations in epigenetic regulators, RHOA and FYN kinase in peripheral T cell lymphomas. Nature Genetics. 2014;**46**(2):166-170

[14] Lemonnier F et al. Recurrent TET2 mutations in peripheral T-cell lymphomas correlate with TFH-like features and adverse clinical parameters. Blood. 2012;**120**(7):1466-1469

[15] Cairns RA et al. IDH2 mutations are frequent in angioimmunoblastic T-cell lymphoma. Blood. 2012;**119**(8): 1901-1903

[16] Crescenzo R et al. Convergent mutations and kinase fusions lead to oncogenic STAT3 activation in anaplastic large cell lymphoma. Cancer Cell. 2015;**27**(4):516-532

[17] Parrilla Castellar ER et al. ALK-negative anaplastic large cell lymphoma is a genetically heterogeneous disease with widely disparate clinical outcomes. Blood. 2014;**124**(9):1473-1480

[18] Wang C et al. IDH2R172 mutations define a unique subgroup of patients with angioimmunoblastic T-cell lymphoma. Blood. 2015;**126**(15): 1741-1752

[19] Amengual JE et al. A phase 1 study of romidepsin and pralatrexate reveals marked activity in relapsed and refractory T-cell lymphoma. Blood. 2018;**131**(4):397-407

[20] Shustov A et al. Romidepsin is effective and well tolerated in older patients with peripheral T-cell lymphoma: Analysis of two phase II trials. Leukemia & Lymphoma. 2017;**58**(10):2335-2341

[21] Cheminant M et al. Efficacy of 5-azacytidine in a TET2 mutated angioimmunoblastic T cell lymphoma. British Journal of Haematology. 2015;**168**(6):913-916

[22] Khwaja A et al. Acute myeloid leukaemia. Nature Reviews. Disease Primers. 2016;**2**:16010

[23] Hood L, Friend SH. Predictive, personalized, preventive, participatory (P4) cancer medicine. Nature Reviews. Clinical Oncology. 2011;**8**(3):184-187

[24] Tsimberidou AM et al. Personalized medicine for patients with advanced cancer in the phase I program at MD Anderson: Validation and landmark analyses. Clinical Cancer Research. 2014;**20**(18):4827-4836

[25] Von Hoff DD et al. Pilot study using molecular profiling of patients' tumors to find potential targets and select treatments for their refractory cancers. Journal of Clinical Oncology. 2010;**28**(33):4877-4883

[26] Le Tourneau C et al. Molecularly targeted therapy based on tumour molecular profiling versus conventional therapy for advanced cancer (SHIVA): A multicentre, open-label, proof-of-concept, randomised, controlled phase 2 trial. The Lancet Oncology. 2015;**16**(13):1324-1334

[27] Irish JM et al. Single cell profiling of potentiated phospho-protein networks in cancer cells. Cell. 2004;**118**(2):217-228

[28] Kornblau SM et al. Dynamic single-cell network profiles in acute myelogenous leukemia are associated with patient response to standard induction therapy. Clinical Cancer Research. 2010;**16**(14):3721-3733

[29] Lacayo NJ et al. Development and validation of a single-cell network profiling assay-based classifier to predict response to induction therapy in paediatric patients with de novo acute myeloid leukaemia: A report from the Children's Oncology Group. British Journal of Haematology. 2013;**162**(2):250-262

[30] Frismantas V et al. Ex vivo drug response profiling detects recurrent sensitivity patterns in drug resistant ALL. Blood. Mar 16, 2017;**129**(11):e26-e37. DOI: 10.1182/blood-2016-09-738070. Epub 2017 Jan 25

[31] Gao D et al. Organoid cultures derived from patients with advanced prostate cancer. Cell. 2014;**159**(1):176-187

[32] van de Wetering M et al. Prospective derivation of a living organoid biobank of colorectal cancer patients. Cell. 2015;**161**(4):933-945

[33] Yu M et al. Cancer therapy. Ex vivo culture of circulating breast tumor cells for individualized testing of drug susceptibility. Science. 2014;**345**(6193):216-220

[34] Hidalgo M et al. Patient-derived xenograft models: An emerging platform for translational cancer research. Cancer Discovery. 2014;**4**(9):998-1013

[35] Roife D et al. Ex vivo testing of patient-derived Xenografts mirrors the clinical outcome of patients with pancreatic ductal adenocarcinoma.

Clinical Cancer Research. 2016;**22**(24):6021-6030

[36] Selby P, Buick RN, Tannock I. A critical appraisal of the "human tumor stem-cell assay". The New England Journal of Medicine. 1983;**308**(3):129-134

[37] Von Hoff DD. Send this patient's tumor for culture and sensitivity. The New England Journal of Medicine. 1983;**308**(3):154-155

[38] Samson DJ et al. Chemotherapy sensitivity and resistance assays: A systematic review. Journal of Clinical Oncology. 2004;**22**(17):3618-3630

[39] Tyner JW et al. Kinase pathway dependence in primary human leukemias determined by rapid inhibitor screening. Cancer Research. 2013;**73**(1):285-296

[40] Andersson EI et al. Discovery of novel drug sensitivities in T-PLL by high-throughput ex vivo drug testing and mutation profiling. Leukemia. 2018;**32**(3):774-787

[41] Boidol B et al. First-in-human response of BCL-2 inhibitor venetoclax in T-cell prolymphocytic leukemia. Blood. 2017;**130**(23):2499-2503

[42] Dearden C. Management of prolymphocytic leukemia. Hematology. American Society of Hematology. Education Program. 2015;**2015**:361-367

[43] Licciardello MP et al. A combinatorial screen of the CLOUD uncovers a synergy targeting the androgen receptor. Nature Chemical Biology. 2017;**13**(7):771-778

[44] He L et al. Patient-customized drug combination prediction and testing for T-cell Prolymphocytic Leukemia patients. Cancer Research. 2018;**78**(9):2407-2418

[45] Fischer U et al. Genomics and drug profiling of fatal TCF3-HLF-positive acute lymphoblastic leukemia identifies recurrent mutation patterns and therapeutic options. Nature Genetics. 2015;**47**(9):1020-1029

[46] Frismantas V et al. Ex vivo drug response profiling detects recurrent sensitivity patterns in drug-resistant acute lymphoblastic leukemia. Blood. 2017;**129**(11):e26-e37

[47] Silva A et al. An ex vivo platform for the prediction of clinical response in multiple myeloma. Cancer Research. 2017;**77**(12):3336-3351

[48] Vladimer GI et al. Global survey of the immunomodulatory potential of common drugs (accepted). Nature Chemical Biology. Jun 2017;**13**(6): 681-690. DOI: 10.1038/nchembio.2360. Epub 2017 Apr 24

[49] Snijder B et al. Image-based ex-vivo drug screening for patients with aggressive haematological malignancies: Interim results from a single-arm, open-label, pilot study. Lancet Haematol. 2017;**4**(12):e595-e606

Chapter 7

Unique Therapeutic Approaches for Targeting Epigenetic Machinery in T-cell Lymphoma

Jacob Cogan and Jennifer E. Amengual

Abstract

Growing knowledge on T-cell lymphoma (TCL) biology has led to the understanding that TCLs harbor derangements in proteins modulating epigenetic control. Some such derangements include mutations in TET2, IDH2, DNMT3A, EP300, and CBP. In addition, overexpression of epigenetic modifiers such as EZH2 also exists in the absence of mutations. HDAC inhibitors are approved for use in relapsed T-cell lymphoma. There may be unique methods to targeting epigenetic derangements using new agents such as DNMT, EZH2, IDH, and BET inhibitors to name a few. In this chapter, we will review and explore unique methods for therapeutic targeting of epigenetic machinery for TCL.

Keywords: T-cell lymphoma, epigenetics, EZH2, DNMT3A, IDH2, TET2, BET, EP300, CBP, DOT1L

1. Introduction

Peripheral T-cell lymphomas (TCL) are a diverse group of non-Hodgkin lymphomas that tend to have aggressive courses and poor prognoses. TCLs account for 10–15% of all non-Hodgkin lymphomas. Common subtypes are anaplastic large cell lymphoma (ALCL), angioimmunoblastic T-cell lymphoma (AITL), cutaneous T-cell lymphoma (CTCL), and peripheral T-cell lymphoma NOS (PTCL-NOS). Even more rare subtypes include adult T-cell leukemia/lymphoma (ATLL) and natural killer/T-cell lymphoma (NKTCL). The diagnosis of these conditions can be challenging, as the largest group of these conditions – PTCL-NOS – cannot currently be further categorized beyond that point [1]. Similarly, the approach to treating TCLs has generally been empiric and homogenous, rather than specific and targeted to the particular subtype.

TCL patients frequently do not respond well to chemotherapy. The median time to relapse or progression after primary therapy was 6.7 months in a sample of 153 patients with PTCL-NOS, AITL, and ALCL, three of the most common TCL subtypes [2]. Further, median overall survival and progression free survival after relapse or progression in this sample was 5.5 and 3.1 months, respectively. Given this poor response to chemotherapy, the subsequent lack of candidacy for stem cell transplantation in most TCL patients given this poor response, and the tendency of TCL patients to develop resistance to chemotherapy, optimal therapies for this population remain undefined. Clinical trials are thus often the recommended first-line treatment for these patients.

Limitations in the specificity of treatment of TCL may be related to prior lack of insight into the genetics and molecular underpinnings of these malignancies. However, as understanding of the genetics of these diseases advances, therapy targeting epigenetic modifiers and transcriptional dysregulation have emerged as a target for TCL therapy [1, 3]. Epigenetic modulators have been found to be widely mutated in TCLs, and are thought to play a central role in these diseases. The heritability of epigenetic profiles across cell lines, and the consistency with which this process is aberrant in TCLs makes targeting epigenetic modifiers an area of promise in treating these particularly resistant conditions [4].

Epigenetics refers to aspects of chromatin biology that affect gene expression without altering DNA sequence. Chromatin is comprised of DNA wrapped around a core of four types of histone proteins, forming nucleosomes. The ability of the transcriptional machinery to access chromatin determines gene expression. This accessibility is determined by posttranslational modifications of the components of the nucleosome complex, such as methylation and acetylation of DNA and histones. Given the inherently plastic and reversible nature of epigenetic modifications, they have emerged as an appealing therapeutic target, in contrast to the more fixed nature of genetic alterations. Further, epigenetic regulators often have enzymatic activities or binding domains that lend themselves well to small molecule inhibition [3].

Epigenetic abnormalities targeted in TCLs tend to be related to methylation and acetylation of histones and DNA. Histone deacetylase (HDAC) inhibitors were the first approved epigenetic therapy for TCL. HDACs tend to be recruited by oncoproteins to support repressive malignant gene expression [3]. The U.S. FDA has approved three HDAC inhibitors for use in relapsed or refractory TCLs. Vorinostat, an oral agent, was approved for relapsed/refractory CTCL in 2006, with romidepsin—an IV agent—following shortly after in 2009 [5]. Romidepsin and belinostat were also approved for the treatment of relapsed/refractory peripheral TCLs 2011 and 2014, respectively. Adverse effects include cytopenias and gastrointestinal symptoms. In addition, romidepsin can lead to EKG changes that may be clinically significant in patients with pre-existing cardiac disease. Interestingly, the clinical benefit derived from HDAC inhibitors in TCLs have not shown the same efficacy

Epigenetic Target	Drug	Cell Line	Reference
EZH2	GSK126	Non-specific TCL	Kumar et al. [25]
	DZNep	ATLL	Daisuke et al. [23]
	DZNep	NKTL	Yan et al. [24]
CBP/EP300	A-485	NHL	Lasko et al. [28]
DOT1L	EPZ-5676	Non-specific TCL	Kumar et al. [30]
DNMT3A	Azacitadine or Decitabine + HDAC inhibitor	CTCL	Marchi et al. [8]
	Decitabine + Chidamide	PTCL-NOS	Ji et al. [26]
	Azacitadine + Romidepsin	Sezary Syndrome	Rozati et al. [7]
	JQ1	CTCL	Kim et al. [40]

Table 1.
Pre-clinical studies of novel epigenetic inhibitors in T-cell lymphoma.

in B-cell lymphomas, further underscoring the importance of pursuing this treatment paradigm for TCLs. Romidepsin, belinostat and vorinostat are currently being studied in combination with conventional chemotherapies [6], such as CHOP [7, 8], gemcitabine [9] and ifosfamide-containing regimens [10].

Given the success of HDAC inhibitors in TCLs, much research has been dedicated towards elucidating other epigenetic targets for TCL therapy (**Tables 1** and **2**). Candidates have included DNA methyltransferases (DNMTs), the ten-eleven

Target	Drug	Phase	Population	Results	Toxicities	Reference
EZH2	DS-3201b	I	5 TCL patients (2 ATLL, 2 AITL, 1 PTCL-NOS)	ORR 80% one CR, three PRs	Hematologic, dysgeusia, diarrhea nasopharyngitis, alopecia, rash, decreased appetite, dry skin	Maruyama et al., [21]
DNMT3A	Azacitadine	I	19 relapsed/ refractory TCL patients (12 AITL)	ORR 53%; 75% ORR for AITL patients, 5 CR	Hematologic, diarrhea	Delarue et al. [31]
	Azacitadine + Romidepsin	I/II	10 TCL patients	ORR 83%, 50% CR	Hematologic, febrile neutropenia	Falchi et al. [32]
IDH2	AG-221	I/II	AITL patients	In progress		NCT02273739

Table 2.
Clinical trials of novel epigenetic inhibitors in T-cell lymphoma.

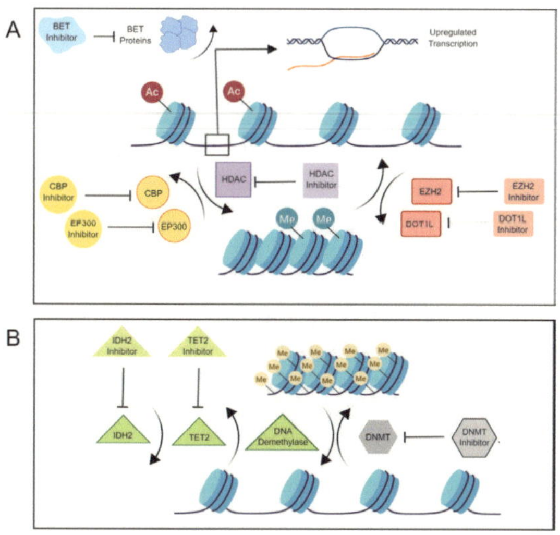

Figure 1.
(A) Histone acetylation makes chromatin more accessible for transcription, while histone deacetylation makes chromatin more compact and less transcriptionally active. Histone acetylation is mediated by histone acetyltransferases, such as CBP and EP300; histone deacetylation is mediated by histone deacetylases (HDACs). Inhibitors of CBP, EP300, and HDACs have all shown promise in treating TCLs. BET proteins recognize acetylated histones and promote transcription at related DNA regions, and can be targeted by BET inhibitors. By contrast, methylation of histones renders DNA transcriptionally inactive, while demethylation of histones increases DNA receptiveness to transcription. EZH2 and DOT1L are histone methylators, and are targets in TCL therapy as well. (B) DNA methylation is associated with transcriptional repression, while de-methylated DNA is more transcriptionally active. TET2 promotes DNA demethylase activity, and IDH2 regulates TET2. TET2 and IDH2 can both be targeted in TCL treatment. Additionally, a major category of TCL therapy involves inhibitor of DNA methyltransferases (DNMTs), which render chromatin more transcriptionally inactive.

translocation (TET) family of proteins, isocitrate dehydrogenase (IDH) enzymes, bromodomain and extra-terminal (BET) proteins, enhancer of zeste homolog 2 (EZH2), cyclic AMP-response element binding, binding protein (CBP) and E1A binding protein p300 (EP300), and disruptor of telomeric silencing 1-like (DOT1L) (**Figure 1**). Further, it has been postulated that combination therapy of different epigenetic modulators may have added utility in TCL treatment. Tumor suppressors are often down regulated by abnormal histone deacetylation and/or DNA methylation. By combining HDAC inhibitors and DNMT inhibitors, synergy may be achieved to relieve this abnormal transcriptional repression [11]. Thus, epigenetic combination therapy may represent a new paradigm for the treatment of TCLs [5, 12]. In this manuscript, we will review the TCL subtypes and relevant documented mutations, survey the literature regarding novel epigenetic therapies for TCL, and discuss future directions for this therapeutic strategy.

2. T-cell lymphoma subtypes

2.1 Anaplastic large cell lymphoma (ALCL)

Anaplastic large cell lymphoma (ALCL) represents up to 32% of TCLs in North America, and about 2.4% of NHLs [5]. It is more common in men (2:1 male: female ratio), and displays a bimodal age distribution, with peaks at age 25 and 60. ALCL frequently involves the lymph nodes or skin, but can also affect the gastrointestinal tract, lung, and bone. Translocations involving the Anaplastic Lymphoma Kinase (ALK) are common in ALCL, with t(2,5) translocations occurring in 50% of cases, and leading to a Nucleophosmin-ALK (NPM-ALK) fusion protein. This protein induces a number of oncogenic signaling pathways, leading to malignant transformation of T-cells [13]. ALK status is important for prognosis, with ALK+ positive displaying a 70% 5-year survival, while ALK-patients have a 49% survival rate [5]. Chemotherapy is the first line treatment for this disease, and crizotinib, an ALK tyrosine kinase inhibitor, can be used in chemotherapy-resistant disease ALK+ ALCL. However, resistance to crizotinib frequently develops, motivating pursuit of other treatment strategies. DNA methylation profiling of five ALCL patients displayed similar patterns of methylation in all samples, regardless of ALK status. This abnormal methylation was noted in genes involved in T-cell differentiation and immune response [14], suggesting a role of epigenetic derangements in driving ALCL development. Inhibitors of BET proteins, which recognize acetylated histones and recruit transcription factors to these regions, have been used in pre-clinical models to treat ALCL, described later in this review.

2.2 Angioimmunoblastic T-cell lymphoma (AITL)

Angioimmunoblastic T-cell lymphoma (AITL) comprises 20% of TCLs and 1% of all NHLs [15]. Patients tend to be diagnosed with advanced stage disease, and have a median survival of less than 3 years. AITLs are unique in their gene expression pattern, with mutations in genes responsible for epigenetic modifications – particularly DNA methylation – emerging as particularly commonplace. In a study of 85 AITL patients, 65 (76%) had TET2 mutations, 43 of which displayed two or three TET2 mutations, indicating strong selective pressure for TET2 abnormalities in AITL. Twenty-eight patients (33%) had DNMT3 mutations, and 17 (20%) had mutations in IDH2. Of note, all but two of the patients in this sample with DNMT3 and IDH2 mutations also had TET2 mutations. Mutations in these specific types of epigenetic modulators are more commonly seen in myeloid malignancies than in other lymphomas. This could help explain the poor outcomes AITL patients have after treatment with chemotherapy regimens developed against BCLs. The multistep tumorigenesis model for AITL hypothesizes that early mutations in epigenetic modifiers interact with late cooperative mutations to enable malignant transformation [5]. As such, TET2, DNMT3, and IDH2, among other epigenetic modulators, have emerged as therapeutic targets in AITL.

2.3 Cutaneous T-cell lymphoma (CTCL)

Cutaneous T-cell lymphoma (CTCL) includes mycosis fungoides (MF), Sezary syndrome (SS), and other related lymphoproliferative disorders that originate in the skin. CTCL is a male-predominant disease (1.7:1.0 M:F ratio), has a median age of diagnosis in the mid-1950s, and is more common in African Americans [5]. MF tends to present with patches, plaques, tumors, and ulcers, while SS presents with exfoliative erythroderma, lymphadenopathy, and circulating Sezary cells. The prognosis of these patients generally correlates with the extent of cutaneous and systemic involvement, with MF displaying an 88% 5-year survival and SS patients demonstrating a 5-year survival of 24%. Currently available therapies have a success rate of 30–50%, and relapses are common [5, 11]. Epigenetics have been important in improving diagnoses of these conditions, with detection of promoter hypermethylation of chemokine-like CMTM2 proving sufficient to distinguish SS from erythrodermic inflammatory dermatosis [16]. As mentioned earlier, CTCL was the first malignancy for which HDAC inhibitors were approved. One such agent, romidepsin, showed an overall response rate (ORR) of 35% and complete response in 6% when used as monotherapy in relapsed/refractory CTCL patients [11]. Currently, a topical HDAC inhibitor for use in early stage CTCL is underway with promising results [17]. There is thought that CTCLs may be susceptible to additional epigenetic modifiers. SS has also been shown to have a high prevalence of methylation abnormalities [4]. TET2 mutations are one of the early genetic abnormalities in SS, and mutations in isocitrate dehydrogenase (IDH) have been described as well [18].

2.4 Adult T-cell leukemia/lymphoma (ATLL)

ATLL is associated with the human T-cell lymphotropic virus-1 (HTLV-1). The virus—endemic to southwestern Japan, the Caribbean, and Central Africa—is transmitted by blood transfusions, needle sharing, sexual intercourse, and breastfeeding. HTLV-1 immortalizes human T-cells, and was the first retrovirus found to be directly associated with malignancy. ATLL occurs in 2.5% of carriers in endemic areas, with growing rates of prevalence in non-endemic areas. Subtypes include smoldering, chronic, lymphoma, and acute ATLL, with 4-year survival rates ranging from 63% for smoldering to 5% for acute. Chemotherapy plus central nervous system prophylaxis is the current first-line treatments for ATLL, with some electing to add antiviral therapy, though virus eradication does not necessarily lead to improved survival [5]. As a result, attention has turned towards understanding the genetic and epigenetic factors involved in causing and maintaining malignant disease in HTLV-1 infected T-cells. ATLL cells display H3K27me3 hypermethylation, a feature mediated by EZH2. EZH2 overexpression leads to this histone hypermethylation, leading to silencing of anti-apoptotic pathways [19]. It is thought that this reprogramming occurs at an early stage of ATLL T-cell development, potentially as a result of the HTLV-1 protein Tax enhancing EZH2 promoter activity. Further, 22% of a 27-patient ATLL cohort were found to have EP300 mutations, with smaller numbers demonstrating mutations in TET2 and DNMT3A [20].

2.5 Natural killer/T-cell lymphoma (NKTL)

Natural killer/T-cell lymphoma (NKTL) constitutes about 11% of TCLs. Prior to the 1990s, the rare disease was known as lethal midline granuloma, in which destructive midline facial lesions would develop, progressing rapidly to cause patient death. Advances in pathology led to recognition that this condition was a neoplasm of lymphoid origin [21]. The disease is predominantly seen in males (2:1 M:F), and the median age of diagnosis is 50 years old. They can be classified as nodal and extranodal, and further as nasal (nose, upper aerodigestive tract; 80% of cases) and non-nasal (skin, GI tract, testes, salivary glands; 20% of cases). Additionally, peripheral blood involvement is common, and further labels the disease as a lymphoma/leukemia subtype. Interestingly, all NKTL lymphoma cells are infected with EBV. Detection of the virus is required for diagnosis, and prognosis can be correlated with EBV levels as time of diagnosis and variation of levels in response to therapy. NKTL is a particularly aggressive condition, with median survival ranging from 12 months for the nasal subtype to 2 months for the lymphoma/leukemia subtype. Concurrent chemoradiation is the mainstay of treatment for NKTL [5], with non-anthracycline based regimens (such as those containing L-asparaginase) proving more effective. While epigenetic therapies have not to this point been utilized in treating NKTL, EP300 and EZH2 mutations have been documented, indicating a possible role for epigenetic therapy in this disease [22].

2.6 Peripheral T-cell lymphoma not otherwise specified (PTCL-NOS)

Peripheral T-cell lymphoma not otherwise specified (PTCL-NOS) constitutes both the largest group of TCLs and the least characterized. PTCL-NOS accounts for 25% of TCLs, and is a diagnosis of exclusion, when the disease does not fit any of the other WHO classifications mentioned above. It tends to affect older men, with a median age of presentation of 60. Nodal disease is common, though any organ can be affected, and about 70% of cases present at advanced stages. PTCL-NOS patients tend to be treated with anthracycline-based chemotherapy regimens. Recurrent mutations in TET2, IDH2, and DNMT3A have been found in the T-follicular helper phenotype of PTCL-NOS. This disease has since been designated as its own entity, distinct from the larger group of PTCL-NOS. Overall, PTCL-NOS patients display an overall survival rate of 32–45%. The HDAC-inhibitors romidepsin and belinostat are approved for relapsed/refractory PTCL-NOS [6].

3. Epigenetic agents targeting histone methylation and acetylation

Epigenetic modification of histones has both documented and emerging therapeutic importance in TCL treatment. Histone acetylation is a dynamic process comprised of acetylation with lysine acetyltransferases and deacetylation with histone deacetylases (HDACs). Acetylation allows for chromatin configurations more accessible to transcription, whereas deacetylation generates more compact, less transcriptionally active chromatin [3]. The importance of HDAC inhibitors have been well documented in TCLs such as CTCL and PTCL-NOS. Transcriptional co-activators such as CBP and EP300 are involved in promoting histone acetylation, and have been targeted in the treatment of ATLL. Histone methylation, by contrast, alters the ability of DNA-reading proteins to bind to methylated residues, while demethylation of histones render associated chromatin more transcriptionally active. EZH2 and DOT1L are clinically important histone methylators, relevant to the treatment of ATLL and NKTL, among other subtypes.

3.1 Enhancer of zeste homolog 2 (EZH2)

Enhancer of zeste homolog 2 (EZH2) is the enzymatic component of polycomb repressor complex 2 (PRC2). PRC2 has documented involvement in cell fate decisions by establishing and maintaining transcriptional repression through post-translational modifications of histones via EZH1 and 2 [23]. EZH2 trimethylates lysine residue 27 of histone H3 (H3K27me3), causing down-regulation of genes involved in tumor suppression and cell differentiation [24]. Elevated levels of H3K27me3 are thought to correlate with the aggressiveness of malignancies such as lymphoma, in addition to brain, breast, kidney, lung, and prostate [25]. While EZH2 is thought to be dispensible for normal hematopoiesis, given it is redundancy with EZH1, EZH2 is the PRC2 component most often implicated in the development of hematological malignancies [3]. EZH2 has emerged as a target for T cell lymphoma therapy. Overexpression of EZH2 has been noted in ATLL [26] and NKTL [27], in particular.

Several pre-clinical studies have demonstrated utility of EZH2 inhibition in T cell lymphoma. GSK126, a commercially available EZH2 inhibitor, was shown to decrease cell viability in an in vitro TCL line [28]. In one study, PTEN-inactivated cells derived from a TCL mouse model were utilized. High concentrations of GSK126 were required to achieve in vitro biological activity, attributed to the high levels of L-amino acid transporter 1 (LAT1) in these cells. As opposed to LAT2, which is expressed in normal cells, LAT1 is predominantly expressed in malignant cells. Such cells with high levels of LAT1 tend to be more resistant to therapeutic treatment, as opposed to cells with lower levels. The authors felt that the high LAT1 levels likely gave the in vitro TCL cells an enhanced ability to combat chemical attacks, via mechanisms such as enhanced essential amino acid sequestering potential. This observation supports their notion that combination therapy will be the most efficacious method to achieving results when using therapies such as EZH2 inhibitors. This point highlights the importance of utilizing combination epigenetic therapies in treating TCLs.

Work performed in our laboratory sought to combine EZH2 and HDAC inhibitors as a means of dual targeting of histone methylation and acetylation. GSK128 was combined with romidepsin across a large panel of lymphoma cells (N-21). Synergy was observed in cell lines with known EZH2 dysregulation including ATLL. We found that the combination led to decreased histone methylation and increased acetylation as compared to treatment with either drug alone. This in turn induced p21 expression leading to caspase 3 and PARP cleavage. The combination is safe and effective in mouse models of lymphoma. Synergy could be predicted in cell lines, which were enriched in chromatin silencing, gene silencing, epigenetic regulation of gene expression and protein acetylation pathways as measured by gene set enrichment analysis (GSEA) [29]. Dual targeting of histone modifications could be a rational approach for diseases driven by epigenetic derangements.

DZNep, an EZH2 inhibitor, has demonstrated pre-clinical efficacy in ATLL and NKTL. In ATLL cell lines, DZNep been shown to deplete levels of both EZH2 and BCL2 [26]. The authors demonstrated that, while untreated ATLL cells demonstrate decreased levels of micro RNA 181a (miR-181a), ATLL cells treated with DZNep showed elevated levels. miR-181a production is modulated by EZH2, and acts as a negative regulator of BCL2 expression. Thus, the inhibitory effects of DZNep on EZH2 results in increased production of miR-181a, decreased levels of BCL2, and consequently apoptosis. Further, in [27], DZNep inhibited growth of NKTL cell lines in an unexpected fashion. These authors noted an oncogenic role of EZH2 independent of its methyltransferase activity. Cells with mutations in EZH2 that depleted their histone methyltransferase activity still had oncogenic potential, likely through increased production of cyclin D1. DZNep was still able to inhibit growth of these cells as well. This indicates that the oncogenicity of EZH2 mutation is more complicated than simply arising through overactive histone methylation, and that therapies should not simply focus on targeting the enzymatic activity of EZH2, but perhaps on the production of EZH2 itself.

In humans, DS-3201b, an oral EZH1/2 dual inhibitor, was utilized in a phase 1 study which included five TCL patients (two ATLL, two AITL, and one PTCL-NOS) [24]. Overall response rate (ORR) in TCL patients was 80%, with one complete response (CR) and three partial responses (PR). ORR in the entire cohort (15 total patients, 10 with other BCLs) was 55%. Adverse events were mainly transient hematologic toxicities.

3.2 Histone acetyltransferases (HATs): CBP/EP300

Cyclic AMP-response element binding, binding protein (CBP) and E1A binding protein p300 (EP300) are highly related transcriptional coactivators, with 75% similarity across their entire length and 63% homology at the amino acid level [19]. They are known to enhance transcription through linking sequence-specific transcription factors to RNA polymerase II. They also facilitate histone acetylation, which promotes transcription. [13]. CBP and EP300 are two of the most frequently mutated histone acetyl transferases in hematologic malignancies [3]. Mutations have been documented in CTCL, ATLL, NKTCL, and PTCL-NOS [1, 3, 20, 30]. They have also been implicated in the actions of viral oncoproteins such as HTLV-1 Tax protein [20]. Acetylation of p53 by CBP has been shown to enhance the DNA binding ability of p53, and loss of CBP has been shown to cause T-cell lymphomagenesis in vitro [31]. In [20], Shah et al. showed that EP300 mutations were present in 22% of a North American cohort of 27 ATLL patients. Five EP300-mutant ATLL cell lines derived from these patients were treated with decitabine, a DNMT-inhibitor. All five lines were sensitive to this treatment, and the addition of doxorubicin demonstrated synergy.

Drug development has focused on small molecule inhibitors of both CBP and EP300. A-485, a combination CBP/EP300 catalytic inhibitor, was evaluated preclinically across a variety of malignant cell lineages. The broadest sensitivity was seen in hematological malignancies, including non-Hodgkin's lymphoma cell lines, with markedly less sensitivity observed in cells derived from solid malignancies [32]. Histone acetyltransferase inhibitors may be of use in treating TCLs via this pathway.

Histone acetyltransferase activators are also in early development. Inactivating mutations in HAT enzymes are monoallelic creating a haploinsufficient state of acetylation. Lymphomas harboring a multitude of epigenetic abnormalities, such as TCLs are poised to capitalize on this relative deficiency. A library of HAT activating compounds have demonstrated efficacy across a panel of lymphoma cell lines and xenograft mouse model [33]. The compounds demonstrated acetylation of histone and p53. In addition, HAT activators demonstrated synergistic cytotoxicity when combined with the HDAC inhibitor, romidepsin. Activating HAT enzymes could therefore be thought of as activating a tumor suppressor and offers a direct method of targeting pathology that drives TCL.

3.3 Disruptor of telomeric silencing 1-like (DOT1L)

Disruptor of telomeric silencing 1-like (DOT1L) is the only known H3 lysine 79 (H3K79) methyltransferase in mammals. Genetic silencing of DOT1L has been shown to impact mitotic spindle formation and cell cycle progression. Preclinical models have shown utility of DOT1L inhibition in AML. Mutations in Mixed-lineage leukemia (MLL) genes, which encode for a family of histone methyltransferases, have been linked to AML (MML1 mutations) and BCLs (MLL2 mutations). The DOT1L containing complex is a frequent translocation partner of MLL fusions in MLL-associated leukemias. Consequently these leukemias have been shown to have atypical H3K79 methylation patterns. Incidentally, AML models carrying recurrent mutations in IDH 1/2 and DNMT3A have also been shown to be susceptible to DOT1L inhibitors. Pinometostat (EPZ-5676), a recently developed DOT1L inhibitor, is currently in phase 1 trials of advanced hematologic malignancies. Given the promising findings of DOT1L inhibition in MLL-associated leukemias, and the efficacy of DOT1L inhibitors in AML models with mutations in epigenetic regulators typical of TCLs, there may be promise in using DOT1L inhibitors in TCLs as well. Thus far, pinometostat has been shown to decrease cell viability in PTEN-inactivated TCL mouse model cells, which have also been utilized in pre-clinical studies of EZH2 inhibitors [3, 34, 35].

4. Epigenetic agents targeting DNA methylation

The regulation and maintenance of DNA methylation plays a key role in cellular differentiation and genome stability. A dynamic process of DNA methylation and demethylation at the carbon-5 position of cytosine nucleotides contributes to the epigenetic milieu of any given cell. DNA methyltransferases such as DNMT3A and DNMT3B are responsible for de novo DNA methylation, while DNMT1 handles maintenance methylation. Conversely, the TET family of proteins handles cytosine demethylation. In contrast to histone acetylation, where an acetylated state leads to more transcriptionally active chromatin, methylated cytosine residues tend to be associated with transcriptional repression. On the other hand, chromatin without cytosine methylation is more transcriptionally active [3]. Abnormalities in DNA methylation have been found to be important in AITL, CTCL, PTCL-NOS, and ALCL.

4.1 DNMT3

DNMT3A, responsible for de novo DNA methylation, is known to be mutated in many hematological malignancies. Azacitidine (5-AZA) and decitabine, two DNMT3A inhibitors, are approved for use in myelodysplastic syndromes and AML. They are nucleoside analogues which incorporate into newly synthesize DNA and RNA strands and subsequently inhibit DNMTs irreversibly. This results in decreased DNA methylation, and consequently, daughter cells likely do not inherit the aberrant methylation pattern. Given the prevalence of DNMT3A mutations in AITL, utilizing DNMT3A inhibitors in this disease has been a focus of much recent research. In a study conducted in France by Delarue [36], 19 patients with relapsed/refractory peripheral TCL were treated with subcutaneously administered 5-AZA. The overall response rate for the entire study population was 55% (10/19). Twelve of the 19 patients had AITL and the ORR for these patients was 75% (9/12). Five of the AITL patients achieved CR, and only 2 of the 9 total responders had experienced progression at the time of analysis. Notably, 8 of the AITL patients had documented TET2 mutations, and all of these patients responded to therapy. 5-AZA treatment elicited no response in 6 of the remaining

7 patients in the study with other TCL subtypes, with the only responder relapsing after cycle 2 of treatment.

PTCL-NOS commonly displays mutations in genes involved in histone methylation and acetylation. The presence of histone modifier gene mutations was associated with decreased progression-free survival in a cohort of 125 PTCL-NOS patients. PTCL-NOS cells were shown to experience growth inhibition when treated with a HDAC inhibitor, chidamide, and decitabine, both in vitro and in vivo [30]. Dual therapy enhanced the interaction of KMT2D with the transcription factor PU.1, consequently inactivating the MAPK, which tends to be constitutively activated in TCL. PU.1 interact with DNMTs to control hematopoiesis and suppress leukemia, and KMT2D is a histone modifier.

Combination therapy involving DMNT3A inhibitors has also shown promise. Transformed CTCL lines were exposed to combination of a DNMT-inhibitor (decitabine or 5-AZA) and an HDAC inhibitor (belinostat, panobinostat, romidepsin, or vorinostat), with induction of apoptosis in all lines treated [12]. Combination therapy with decitabine and belinostat also induced significant growth delay in an in vivo mouse model, compared to mice treated with single agent therapy. Gene expression analysis showed that, as opposed to the 138 genes modulated by romidepsin monotherapy, combination therapy led to modulation of an additional 390 genes, with many involved in apoptosis and cell cycle arrest. These findings further elucidate the molecular basis of the synergism elicited by combination therapy.

Another study utilized a combination of romidepsin and 5-AZA in cell lines from SS patients. Synergistic antiproliferative effects and induction of apoptosis were observed with combination therapy. The concentration of each agent in the combination was 50% less than the IC50 of each when used individually, which may result in improved tolerability when these agents are used clinically [11].

Building off these results, in [37], Falchi et al. presented a phase 1/2 trial with combination therapy of romidepsin and 5-AZA in the treatment of lymphoma patients. 10/30 patients in the study had TCLs. While the ORR for all 25 cohort patients evaluable for efficacy was 28% (7/25), with a 16% CRR (4/25), the 6 evaluable TCL patients demonstrated an 83% ORR (5/6) and a 50% CRR (3/6). Combination therapy was generally well tolerated: 5 dose limiting toxicities were recorded, including neutropenia (2), thrombocytopenia (1), pleural effusion (1), and a missed dose (1). Five total patients experienced thrombocytopenia, with three experiencing febrile neutropenia.

4.2 TET2

The ten-eleven translocation (TET) family of proteins are dioxygenases which catalyze DNA demethylation [38]. Aberrant demethylation has been linked to dysregulation of molecules such as BCL6, the transcription factor involved in the differentiation of T helper cells [39]. Abnormal differentiation of these cells provides opportunities for them to obtain late cooperative mutations rendering them malignant. TET2 mutations are frequently seen in mature TCLs [3]. In a study evaluating 190 TCL patients for TET2 mutations, 40/86 (47%) AITL patients carried the mutation, as did 22/58 (38%) PTCL-NOS patients. No other forms of TCL carried the mutation in this sample (18 ALCL patients and 12 NKTL patients, among others). TET2 mutations have been shown to occur in up to 80% of AITL patients [23]. TET2 mutations are also associated with advanced disease and shorter progression free survival.

The development of TET2 inhibitors for TCLs is currently in pre-clinical stages. TCL patients with TET2 mutations frequently also display mutations in RHOA, a GTP-ase important in stem cell differentiation, cell migration and cell shape. The cooperation of these two mutations in TCL progression, and whether small molecule inhibitors can halt or reverse disease progression, is under investigation [40].

4.3 IDH2

Changes in DNA methylation can occur indirectly, as a consequence of mutation of isocitrate dehydrogenase (IDH) enzymes. IDH2 is a regulator of TET2, and mutations in IDH2 have been described in up to 45% of patients with AITL [3]. Biochemically, IDH2 catalyzes the conversion of isocitrate to 2-oxoglutarate (2OG). In AITL, mutant IDH2 generates (R)-2-hydroxyglutarate (2HG), an oxymetabolite potentially contributing to malignant transformation through inhibition of 2OG-dependent enzymes. These enzymes are involved in functions ranging from DNA and histone modification to cellular differentiation, thus primed to produce malignancy when abnormally regulated. AG-221, a, orally available small molecule inhibitor of IDH2, has been tested in phase 1 and 2 trials of patients with AITL and AML (NCT02273739) [3, 39]. Given the frequent co-occurrence of IHD2 and TET2 mutations, combination therapy with inhibitors of each may have promise [41].

4.4 Bromodomain and extra-terminal (BET)

Bromodomain and extra-terminal (BET) proteins play a role in epigenetic memory and regulation of growth-promoting gene transcription [42]. BRD2, BRD3, BRD4, and testis-specific BRDT recognize acetylated lysine residues on histone tails and recruit transcriptional regulatory complexes to facilitate transcription of genes involved in cell cycle progression and apoptosis [43]. For instance, BRD4 regulates MYC transcription. OTX015, an oral BRD2/3/4 inhibitor, induced cell cycle arrest in 5/8 ALCL cell lines. ALK status had no impact on likelihood of response. OTX015 was found to suppress the transcription of the MYC gene in 4/4 cell lines [44].

Amplifications of the MYC oncogene are common in CTCL, occurring in 42.5% of leukemic CTCLs. JQ1, a selective small molecule inhibitor of BET proteins, dose-dependently decreased the cell number of CTCL cells through G1 cell cycle arrest and down-regulation of c-MYC expression. It also inhibited tumor growth of CTCL cells in vivo [45]. Several other types of BET inhibitors have been shown to induce dose-dependent decreases in viability of nine CTCL cell lines, and combining BET inhibitors with HDAC inhibitors potentiated this effect. Importantly, combination therapy was effective in cell lines from patients previously treated with other single therapies, including prior romidepsin monotherapy with relapse in one cell line. Significant reduction of BCL2 and MYC expression was seen in cells treated with combination therapy. Given that there is a 25% overlap in genes induced by BET inhibitors and HDAC inhibitors separately, it is theorized that the synergy of this combination therapy lies in the induction of HDAC-silenced genes, enabled by BET inhibition. Initial MYC amplification status was not found to be predictive of sensitivity to BET inhibition or the synergy of therapies used in combination. Finally, a functional interdependence between BRD4 and DOT1L in specific types of transcriptional regulation has been noted, suggesting a possible role for combination therapy involving inhibitors of these two molecules [3].

4.5 Anti-fols

The vitamin folate is essential as a source of the one carbon group required to methylate DNA. The folate pathway, and thus the 1-carbon pathway and DNA methylation is complex, built within it many checks and balances to maintain normal DNA methylation. Low folate status induced by diet or drugs can have "destabilizing consequences," resulting in impaired production of thymidine leading to uracil insertion in the DNA sequence, global DNA hypomethylation and ultimately chromosome instability and breakage.

There are two forms of folate that can enter the body depending on the mode of consumption. Folate comes from natural food sources, and folic acid comes from supplements or fortified foods. When folate enters the cell, it is metabolized to 5-methyl-tetrahydrofoate (5-methyl THF). Folic acid however is first reduced to dihydrofolate by dihydrofolate reductase and then to tetrahydrofolate (THF). Polyglutamination of THF allows for cellular retention. After a series of steps, THF is converted to 5-methyl-THF [46]. 5-Methyl THF is then converted to methionine and back to THF by methionine synthase which acts as the 1-carbon donor for S-adenosylmethionine (SAM). SAM donates methyl groups to DNA via DNMT1, 3a, and 3b. We have discussed the role of DNMT inhibitors as effective therapy for TCLs and will now focus on inhibition of other pathways as a means of decreasing DNA methylation (**Figure 2**).

Methotrexate is a widely used antimetabolite utilized as an antineoplastic agent since the 1950s [47, 48]. It has been used for the treatment of CTCL and other T-cell lymphoproliferative disorders such as lymphomatoid papulosis. Patients are often treated with low doses in a metronomic fashion. Methotrexate is a folic acid analogue and one of its actions is to block dihydrofolate reductase which disrupts the folic acid pathway. Evaluation in CTCL cell lines treated with methotrexate led to a decrease in SAM and subsequently decreased promoter region methylation leading to increase FAS protein expression. The addition of SAM was able to overcome the effects induced by methotrexate. Methotrexate, however, has not had the same success in the treatment of the more aggressive PTCL.

Pralatrexate is not merely a second-generation methotrexate. Although, similar to methotrexate, pralatrexate exerts its effects by inhibition of DHFR, it has higher affinity for the reduced folate carrier-1 (RFC-1) and has greater cellular retention through high a rate of forming polyglutamylated conjugates [49]. RFC-1 is an oncofetal protein expressed mostly on the membranes of fetal and tumor cells. This allows some selectivity of pralatrexate for malignant cells over normal cells. Interestingly, pralatrexate has enhanced activity in TCL and to date across several clinical studies, the only B-cell lymphoma that has demonstrated sensitivity to pralatrexate is follicular lymphoma. TCLs and follicular lymphoma biology's share the common feature of increased methylation of DNA and histone. One potential mechanism of action of pralatrexate, may be through modulation of methylation. Though not well

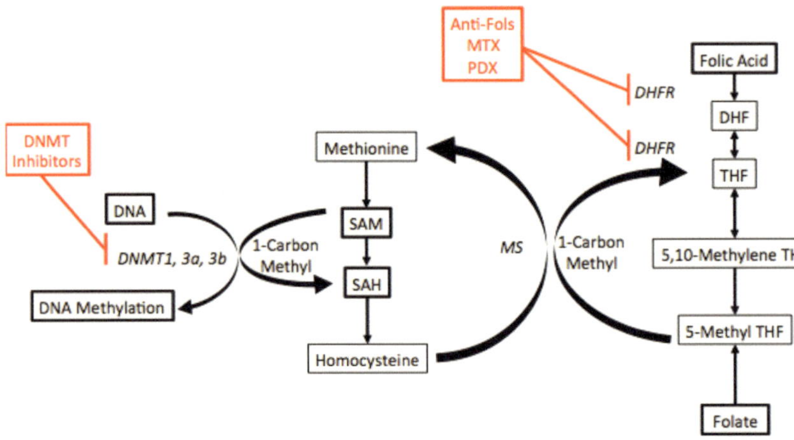

Figure 2.
Direct and indirect inhibition of DNA methylation. DNA methylation can be inhibited directly by inhibiting the DNMT enzymes with DNMT inhibitors azacitidine and decitabine. DNA methylation may be inhibited indirectly by decreasing the 1-carbon methyl donor pool. This can be accomplished via treatment with methotrexate or pralatrexate. Key: MTX, methotrexate; PDX, pralatrexate; DHF, dihydrofolate; THF, tetrahydrofolate; DHFR, dihydrofolate reductase; MS, methionine synthase; SAM, S-adenosylmethionine; SAH, S-adenosylhomocysteine; DNMT, DNA methyltransferase.

understood, by inhibiting DHFR, the 1-carbon pathway may be disrupted. We have observed in our laboratory that treatment of TCL cell lines with pralatrexate does in fact lead to decreased SAM and increased SAH depleting the pool of 1-carbon methyl donors (unpublished data). These initial studies merit further investigation to validate whether this translates into modulation of DNA methylation.

Clinically, the combination of pralatrexate and romidepsin demonstrated an early signal of response for patient with TCL treated on a phase I clinical study [50]. Of the 14 patients with TCL that were evaluable for response, 10 (71%) achieved a response with a complete response rate achieved in 4/10 and a partial response in 6/10 patients. Of the B-cell lymphoma patients only those with follicular lymphoma responded, with 3/4 follicular lymphomas achieving a partial remission. This combination may be acting as a dual epigenetic therapy of sorts, with pralatrexate serving as the hypomethylating agent and romidepsin as the HDAC inhibitor. Thinking about anti-fols in this way, we may come to a new understanding of how to better utilize these old drugs (such as methotrexate) for new purposes.

5. Conclusion

As our understanding of the pathologic drivers of distinct subtypes of TCL grows, we are learning that epigenetic derangements play an important role in lymphomagenesis. Some such derangements include mutations in TET2, IDH2, DNMT3A, EP300, and CBP. Collectively these mutations contribute to a chromatin silenced and chemo-resistant state. In the 10 years since the approval of HDAC inhibitors for TCL, there has been a burst in the creation of novel agents and the repurposing of others to target such biology in TCL. Many of these agents are already being studied in the clinical setting and the clinical application of these agents in TCL is beginning to be realized. The next steps will involve finding the most safe and effective combinations that will best induce durable complete responses. These agents might be best utilized for discrete TCL subtypes, for example DNMT inhibitors for AITL and EZH2 inhibitors for ATLL. Furthermore, as we now have an understanding that epigenetics is crucial to the development of these lymphomas, we need to understand how this intersects with immune function and the microenvironment as well as the metabolic disposition of these malignant cells. Answering some of these questions will enable finding the right partners for these drugs whether it be PI3K inhibitors, PD1 inhibitors or BCL2 mimetics. As the field of targeted therapy for TCL grows, we now have the opportunity to supplant the ineffective chemotherapy based treatment for TCL.

Author details

Jacob Cogan and Jennifer E. Amengual*
Center for Lymphoid Malignancies, Columbia University Medical Center, New York, United States

*Address all correspondence to: jea2149@columbia.edu

References

[1] Moffitt AB, Dave SS. Clinical applicaations of the genomic landscape of aggressive non-Hodgkin lymphoma. Journal of Clinical Oncology. 2017;**35**(9):955-963. DOI: 10.1200/JCO.2016.71.7603

[2] Mak V, Hamm J, Chhanabhai M, Shenkier T, Klasa R, Sehn LH, et al. Survival of patients with peripheral T-cell lymphoma after first relapse or progression: Spectrum fo disease and rare long-term survivors. Journal of Clinical Oncology. 2013;**31**:1970-1976. DOI: 10.1200/JCO.2012.44.7524

[3] Gallipoli P. Seminars in Cancer Biology. 2017. DOI: 10.1016/j.semcancer.2017.07.005

[4] Whittaker S. Global patterns of methylation in Sezary syndrome provide insight into the role of epigenetics in cutaneous T-cell lymphoma. Journal of Investigative Dermatology. 2016;**136**:1753-1754. DOI: 10.1016/j.jid.2016.05.114

[5] Ma H, Abdul-Hay M. T-cell lymphomas, a challenging disease: Types, treatments, and future. International Journal of Clinical Oncology. 2017;**22**:18-51. DOI: 10.1007/s10147-016-1045-2

[6] Broccoli A, Zinzani PL. Review article: Peripheral T-cell lymphoma, not otherwise specified. Blood. 2017;**129**:1103-1112. DOI: 10.1182/blood-2016-08-692566

[7] Dupuis J, Morschhauser F, Ghesquieres H, Tilly H, Casanovas O, Thieblemont C, et al. Combination of romidepsin with cyclophosphamide, doxorubicin, vincristine, and prednisone in previously untreated patients with peripheral T-cell lymphoma: A non-radomised, phase 1b/2 study. Lancet Haematology. 2015;**2**(4):e160-e165. DOI: 10.1016/S2352-3026(15)00023-X

[8] Johnston PB, Cashen AF, Nikolinakos PG, Beaven AW, Barta SK, Bhat G, et al. Safe and effective treatment of patients with peripheral T-cell lymphoma with the novel HDAC inhibitor, belinostat, in combination with CHOP: Results of the Bel-CHOP phase 1 trial. Blood. 2015;**126**:253

[9] Pelligrini C, Dodero A, Chiappella A, Monaco F, Deg'Innocenti D, Salvi F, et al. Italian Lymphoma Foundation: A phase II study on the role of gemcitabine plus romidepsin (GEMRO regimen) in the treatment of relapsed/refractory peripheral T-cell lymphoma patients. Journal of Hematology and Oncology. 2016;**9**:38. DOI: 10.1186/s13045-016-0266-1

[10] Strati P, Chihara D, Oki Y, Fayad LE, Fowler N, Nastoupil L, et al. A phase I study of romidepsin and ifosfamide, carboplatin, etoposide for the treatment of patients with relapsed of refractory peripheral T-cell lymphoma. Haematologica. 2018;**103**(9):e416-e418. DOI: 10.3324/haematol.2018.187617

[11] Rozati S, Kim YH. Experimental treatment strategies in primary cutaneous T-cell lymphomas. Current Opinion Oncology. 2016;**28**(2):166-171. DOI: 10.1097/CCO.0000000000000272

[12] Marchi E, Zullo KM, Amengual JE, Kalac M, Bongero D, McIntosh CM, et al. The combination of hypomethylating agents and histone deacetylase inhibitors produce marked synergy in preclinical models of T-cell lymphoma. British Journal of Haematology. 2015;**171**:215-226. DOI: 10.1111/bjh.13566

[13] Scheifer AI, Vesely P, Hassler MR, Egger G, Kenner L. The role of AP-1

and epigenetics in ALCL. Frontiers in Bioscience. 2015;7:226-235

[14] Hassler MR, Pulverer W, Lakshminarasimhan R, Weinhaeusel A, Turner SD, Egger G. Insights into the pathogenesis of anaplastic large-cell lymphoma through genome-wide DNA methylation profiling. Cell Reports. 2016;**17**(2):596-608. DOI: 10.1016/j.celrep.2016.09.018

[15] Odejide O, Weigert O, Lane AA, Toscano D, Lunning MA, Kopp N, et al. A targeted mutational landscape of angioimmunoblastic T-cell lymphoma. Blood. 2014;**123**(9):1293-1296. DOI: 10.1182/blood-2013-10-531509

[16] van Doorn R, Slieker RC, Boonk SE, Zoutman WH, Goeman JJ, Bagot M, et al. Epigenetic analysis of Sezary syndrome define patterns of aberrant DNA methylation and identifies diagnostic markers. Journal of Investigative Dermatology. 2016;**136**:1876-1884. DOI: 10.1016/j.jid.2016.03.042

[17] Duvic M, Kim YH, LeBoeuf NR, Porcu P, Hastings J, Bassuner J, et al. A phase 2 randomized study of SHAPE gel (SHP-141) in patients with early-stage cutaneous T-cell lymphoma: Interim results. Journal of Clinical Oncology. 2016;**34**(15):7562. DOI: 10.1200/JCO.2016.34.15_suppl.7562

[18] Cyrenne BM, Lewis J, Weed J, Carlson K, Mirza FN, Foss F, et al. Synergy of BCL2 and histone deacetylase inhibition against leukemic cells from cutaneous T-cell lymphoma patients. Blood. 2017;**130**(19):2073-2083. DOI: 10.1182/blood-2017-06-792150

[19] Fujikawa D, Nakagawa S, Hori M, Kurokawa N, Soejima A, Nakano K, et al. Polycomb-dependent epigenetic landscape in adult T-cell lymphoma. Blood. 2016;**127**(14):1790-1802. DOI: 10.1182/blood-2015-08-662593

[20] Shah UA, Chung EY, Giricz O, Pradhan K, Kataoka K, Gordon-Mitchell S, et al. North American ATLL has a distinct mutational and transcriptional profile and responds to epigenetic therapies. Blood. 2018;**132**(14):1507-1518. DOI: 10.1182/blood-2018-01-824607

[21] Tse E, Kwong YL. The diagnosis and management of NK/T-cell lymphomas. Journal of Hematology Oncology. 2017;**10**(1):85. DOI: 10.1186/s13045-017-0452-9

[22] Zhang Y, Li C, Xue W, Zhang M, Li Z. Frequent mutations in natural killer/T-cell lymphoma. Cell Physiology and Biochemistry. 2018;**49**(1):1-16. DOI: 10.1159/000492835

[23] Roy DM, Walsh LA, Chan TA. Driver mutations of cancer epigenomes. Protein and Cell. 2014;**5**(4):265-296. DOI: 10.1007/s13238-014-0031-6

[24] Maruyama D, Tobinai K, Makita S, Ishida T, Kusumoto S, Ishitsuka K, et al. First-in-human study of the EZH1/2 dual inhibitor DS-3201b in patients with relapsed or refractory non-Hodgkin lymphomas–Preliminary results. Blood. 2017;**130**:4070

[25] Yamagishi M, Uchimaru K. Targeting EZH2 in cancer therapy. Current Opinion in Oncology. 2017;**29**:375-381. DOI: 10.1097/CCO.0000000000000390

[26] Daisuke S, Hiroo H, Hiroaki T, Imaizumi Y, Naoki U, Yoshitomo M, et al. EZH2 inhibitor DZNep induces apoptosis in adult T-cell leukemia/lymphoma cells by BCL2 suppression via regulation of Mir-181a. Blood. 2013;**122**:4265

[27] Yan J, Ng SB, Liang-Seah J, Lin B, Koh TL, Tan J, et al. EZH2 overexpression in natural killer/T-cell lymphoma confers growth advantage independently of histone

methyltransferase activity. Blood. 2013;**121**(22):4512-4520. DOI: 10.1182/blood-2012-08-450494

[28] Kumar A, Kumar V, Lightner JW, Little AL, Jutabha P, Endou H, et al. EZH2 inhibitor GSK126 for cancer treatment: Metabolism, drug transporter and rat pharmacokinetic studies. Medical Research Archives. 2015;**SI**(3). Available from: https://www.journals.ke-i.org/index.php/mra/article/view/273

[29] Lue JK, Prahbu SA, Liu Y, Verma A, Elemento O, Amengual JE. Dual inhibition of EZH2 and HDAC is synergistic in EZH2 dysregulated lymphomas. Hematological Oncology. 2017;**35**(S2):254-255

[30] Ji MM, Huang YH, Huang JY, Wang ZF, Fu D, Liu H, et al. Histone modified gene mutations in peripheral T-cell lymphoma not otherwise specified. Haematologica. 2018;**103**:679-687. DOI: 10.3324/haematol.2017/182444

[31] Kang-Decker N, Tong C, Boussouar F, Baker DJ, Xu W, Leontovich AA, et al. Loss of CBP causes T cell lymphomagenesis in synergy with p27Kip1 insufficiency. Cancer Cell. 2004;**5**(2):177-189

[32] Lasko LM, Jakob CG, Edaji RP, Qiu W, Montgomery D, Digiammarino EL, et al. Discovery of a potent catalytic p300-CBP inhibitor that targets lineage-specific tumors. Nature. 2017;**550**(7674):128-132. DOI: 10.1038/nature24028

[33] Liu Y, Fiorito J, Gonzalez Y, Zuccarello E, Calcagno E, Mazzeo A, et al. Development of First-in-Class Histone Acetyltransferase Activators for Precision Targeting of Epigenetic Derangements in Lymphoma. In: American Society of Hematology Annual Meeting: Oral Presentation; 2018. Available from: https://ash.confex.com/ash/2018/webprogram/Paper110447.html

[34] Stein EM, Garcia-Manero G, Rizzieri DA, Tibes R, Berdeja JG, Savona MR, et al. The DOT1L inhibitor pinometostat reduces H3K79 methylation and has modest clinical activity in adult acute leukemia. Blood. 2018;**131**(240):2661-2669. DOI: 10.1182/blood-2017-12-818948

[35] Kumar V, Kumar A, Lightner JW, Rice PJ, Nebout M, Peyron JF, et al. DOT1L inhibitor EPZ-5676: Synthesis, pharmacokinetic and tissue distribution studies in Sprague-Dawley rats. Medical Research Archives. 2015;**3**

[36] Delarue R, Dupuis J, Sujobert P, Barbieux S, Marcais A, Tournilhac O, et al. Treatment with hypomethylating agent 5-Azacytidine induces sustained response in angioimmunoblastic T-cell lymphomas. Blood. 2016;**128**:4164

[37] Falchi L, Lue JK, Amengual JE, Sawas A, Deng C, Marchi E, et al. A phase ½ study of oral 5-Azacitadine and Romidepsin in patients with lymphoid malignancies reveals promising activity in heavily pretreated peripheral T-cell lymphoma. Blood. 2017;**130**:1515

[38] Lemmonier F, Couronne L, Parrens M, Jais JP, Travert M, Lamant L, et al. Recurrent TET2 mutations in peripheral T-cell lymphomas correlate with TFH-like features and adverse clinical parameters. Blood. 2012;**120**(7):1455-1459. DOI: 10.1182/blood-2012-02-408542

[39] Willemsen M, Schouten HC. Inappropriate costimulation and aberrant DNA methylation as therapeutic targets in angioimmunoblastic T-cell lymphoma. Biomarker Research. 2017;**5**:6. DOI: 10.1186/s40364-017-0085-8

[40] Rao A. Novel Therapeutic Strategies for Peripheral T-Cell Lymphoma by Targeting TET2. 2014. Available from: https://www.lls.org/content/

novel-therapeutic-strategies-for-peripheral-t-cell-lymphoma-by-targeting-tet2-and-rhoa [Accessed: October 25, 2018]

[41] Rodriguez-Cortes J, Palomero T. The curious origins of angioimmunoblastic T-cell lymphoma. Current Opinion in Hematology. 2016;**23**(4):434-443. DOI: 10.1097/MOH.0000000000000261

[42] Jagadeesh D, Smith MR. Novel targeted therapies in peripheral T cell lymphoma. Disoveries in Medicine. 2013;**15**(85):367-378

[43] Kamijo H, Sugaya M, Takahashi N, Oka T, Miyagaki T, Asano Y, et al. BET bromodomain inhibitor JQ1 decreases CD30 and CCR4 expression and proliferation of cutaneous T-cell lymphoma cell lines. Archives of Dermatology Research. 2017;**309**(6): 491-497. DOI: 10.1007/s00403-017-1749-9

[44] Boi M, Bonetti P, Ponzoni M, Tibiletti MG, Stahis A, Cvitkovic E, et al. The Brd-inhibitor OTX015 shows pre-clinical activity in anaplastic large T-cell lymphoma (ALCL). Blood. 2012;**120**:4872

[45] Kim SR, Lewis JM, Cyrenne BM, Monico PF, Mirza FN, Carlson KR, et al. BET inhibition in advanced cutaneous T cell lymphoma is synergistically potentiated by BCL2 inhibition or HDAC inhibition. Oncotarget. 2018;**9**(49):29193-29207. DOI: 10.18632/oncotarget.25670

[46] Crider KS, Yang TP, Berry RJ, Bailey LB. Folate and DNA menthylation: A review of molecular mechanisms and the evidence for folate's role. Advances in Nutrition. 2012;**3**(1):21-38. DOI: 10.3945/an.111.000992

[47] Wood GS, Wu J. Methotrexate and pralatrexate. Dermatologic Clinics. 2015;**33**(4):747-755. DOI: 10.1016/j.det.2015.05.009

[48] Wu J, Wood GS. Reduction of Fas/CD95 promoter methylation, upregulation of Fas protein, and enhancement of sensitivity to apoptosis in cutaneous T-cell lymphoma. Archives of Dermatological Research. 2011;**147**(4):443-449. DOI: 10.1001/archdematol.2010.376

[49] Izbicka E, Diaz A, Streeper R, Wick M, Campos D, Steffen R, et al. Distinct mechanistic activity profile of pralatrexate in comparison to other antifolates in in vitro and in vivo models of human cancers. Cancer Chemotherapy and Pharmacology. 2009;**64**(5):993-999. DOI: 10.1007/s00280-009-0954-4

[50] Amengual JE, Lichtenstein R, Lue J, Sawas A, Deng C, Lichtenstein E, et al. A phase 1 study of romidepsin and pralatrexate reveals marked activity in relapsed and refractory T-cell lymphoma. Blood. 2018;**131**(4):397-407. DOI: 10.1182/blood-2017-09-806737

Chapter 8

Novel Aurora Kinase Inhibitor-Based Combination Therapies for PTCL

Pavan Tenneti, Lisa E. Davis and Daruka Mahadevan

Abstract

Peripheral T-cell lymphomas (PTCLs) are a rare, heterogeneous group of T-cell non-Hodgkin's lymphomas (T-NHL) that display distinct clinical and biological features. Despite a detailed understanding of PTCL transformation, there is no current accepted standard of care for newly diagnosed or relapsed/refractory (r/r) patients. PTCL are highly proliferative neoplasms with an immunosuppressive microenvironment that elaborates drug resistance to current therapies with poor outcomes. Aurora kinases (AKs) are a family of mitotic oncogenic serine/threonine kinases (A, B/C) that are aberrantly expressed in PTCL, providing a growth advantage. Alisertib, an AK-A inhibitor, blocks the mitotic phase of the cell cycle resulting in apoptosis. Preclinical and clinical trials in PTCL demonstrated an ~30% response rate in r/r PTCL similar to other investigational agents. In order to improve response rates, alisertib-based combination therapies were tested with HDAC inhibitors, romidepsin and vorinostat, in phase Ib trials. To improve response rates to alisertib, we evaluated alisertib-induced polyploidy as a drug resistance mechanism by targeting microtubules with vincristine. In addition, we also targeted immunosuppression-induced proliferation with an anti-PD-L1 antibody and PI3K inhibition in PTCL. Targeting aberrant proliferation and immunosuppression is a novel strategy that warrants evaluation in clinical trials for PTCL, an unmet clinical need.

Keywords: peripheral T-cell lymphoma, aurora kinases, aurora kinase inhibitors, immune therapy, targeted therapy

1. Introduction

Peripheral T-cell lymphoma (PTCL) is a heterogeneous group of lymphoproliferative disorders that comprise ~10% of non-Hodgkin's lymphomas (NHL) [1]. PTCL is classified into at least 19 different subtypes affecting precursor T cells or mature post-thymic T cells with the cell of origin, an activated memory CD44+ T cell [2]. Approximately 60% of PTCL diagnoses fall into one of the four subtypes [e.g., peripheral T-cell lymphoma not otherwise specified (PTCL-NOS, 26%), anaplastic large-cell lymphoma (ALCL, ALK+ 7%, ALK- 6%), angioimmunoblastic T-cell lymphoma (AITL, 19%), and enteropathy T-cell lymphoma (<5%)] [3]. Frontline anthracycline-based therapies (e.g., CHOP-like) utilized in diffuse large B-cell lymphoma (DLBCL) provide inferior outcomes to PTCL (NOS) and ALCL-ALK- versus ALCL-ALK+ disease [4]. Further, for CD30+ PTCL (19/26

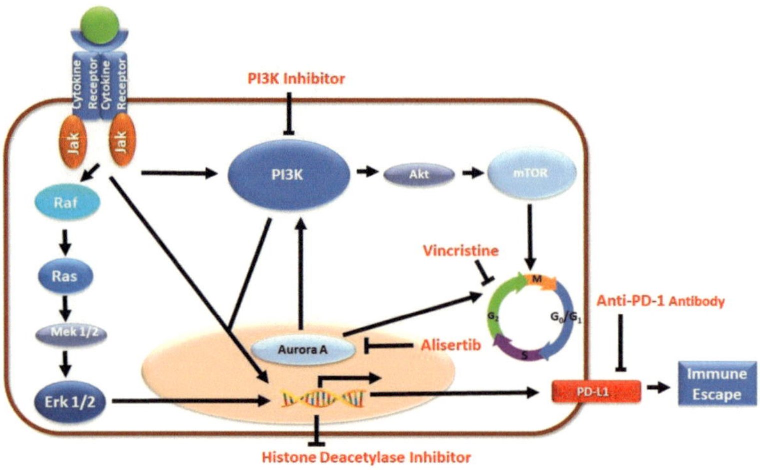

Figure 1.
Aurora kinase-based combination therapy for PTCL (modified from Mahadevan et al. [63]). Inhibition of aurora A kinase (e.g., alisertib) activates PI3K signaling in PTCL which in turn enhances the induction of PD-L1. Cytokine signaling through the MAPK pathway also induces PD-L1 expression leading to profound immune suppression in PTCL. Targeting mitosis with alisertib and immune suppression with an anti-PD-L1 antibody leads to a highly synergistic combination in a syngeneic mouse model of PTCL [52]. Targeting mitosis with alisertib plus vincristine is synergistic causing mitotic catastrophe. This combination is synthetic lethal when combined with anti-PD-L1 plus PI3K inhibition [52]. Further, Aurora A kinase inhibition combined with histone deacetylase inhibitors is also synergistic implicating epigenetic modulation.

ALCL), frontline brentuximab vedotin + CHP had a 92% complete response rate with an estimated 5-year PFS and OS rates of 52 and 80%, respectively, suggestive of an treatment option that is curative for some patients with CD30+ PTCL [5]. In addition, for young fit chemosensitive patients in the relapse setting, HD therapy followed by auto-SCT may be curative in a small proportion of patients [6].

PTCL patients with refractory or relapsed disease should be encouraged to participate in clinical trials with novel investigational agents [7]. USFDA has approved four drugs as single agents: pralatrexate (an antifolate), romidepsin and belinostat (histone deacetylase [HDAC] inhibitors), and brentuximab vedotin (anti-CD30 Mab-ADC). Several agents have demonstrated antitumor activity with response rates of 10–30% (e.g., gemcitabine, bendamustine, duvelisib, copanlisib, alisertib, mogamulizumab) [8]. Preclinical studies with novel agents support combinations that target cell proliferation and immune suppression which are expected to enhance degree, depth, and duration of responses in PTCL. Here, we review novel aurora kinase inhibitor-based combination therapies for PTCL (**Figure 1**).

2. Aurora kinases

The aurora kinases (Aks) are a family of serine/threonine kinases that regulates multiple aspects of cell division and proliferation through the mitotic (M) phase of the cell cycle. They play an essential role in progression through the cell cycle during mitosis and meiosis in ensuring error-free chromosome arrangement around assembly of the mitosis spindle, centrosome alignment and separation, and cytokinesis [9–12]. AKs are composed of three highly conserved isoforms, aurora A, B, and C, which share substantial similarity in sequence and structure in their catalytic domain but are diverse in N-terminal domain sequence, subcellular localization, and functions [13, 14]. AKs A and B are ubiquitously expressed in normal tissues, whereas AK C is specifically expressed in the testis, where it functions primarily in spermatogenesis [13, 15]. AK A localizes primarily at centrosomes, spindle poles, and later on the spindle midzone, where it recruits the cyclin B1-CDK1 complex and promotes the cell to mitotic entry and exit, centrosome separation and maturation, and bipolar spindle assembly [9, 11, 16–18]. Inhibition of AK A causes defects in chromosome segregation and maturation, mitotic spindle aberrations, non-diploidy, cell cycle arrest, and apoptosis [15, 19, 20].

AK B is referred to as a chromosomal passenger protein and, along with other regulatory proteins, constitutes the chromosome passenger complex [13, 15, 16]. This complex concentrates at centrosomes and the central spindle, then relocalizes to the midzone to ensure proper chromosome alignment and segregation and spindle assembly, and regulates cytokinesis [12, 13, 15, 16]. Inhibition of AK B interferes with normal chromosomal alignment during mitosis and leads to inhibition of histone H3 phosphorylation, cytokinesis failure, and polyploidization [15, 21].

AK C concentrates in the centrosomes and shares interacting proteins and functional overlap with AK B during mitosis, although its primary role is in meiosis, where it is necessary for efficient spermatogenesis [22]. With similar structural and localization properties, its functions may be redundant or cooperative to those of AK B [22].

2.1 Role of aurora kinases in tumorigenesis

AKs A and B are frequently amplified in many epithelial tumors, cancers of solid organs, and hematological malignancies, with elevated levels of mRNA and protein present in tumors [11, 19]. Amplification of the chromosomal region that encodes *AURKA* has been linked to high levels of expression of AK A in a wide range of tumor types, and strong expression of the *AURKB* gene is observed in many tumor types [20]. AK A overexpression is sufficient to transform NIH/3T3 cells in vitro, which then induced tumors when transplanted into nude mice [12]. In addition, increased risk of breast, non-small cell lung, esophageal, and ovarian cancer is associated with the *AURKA* Phe31Ile polymorphism [18]. Furthermore, aberrant AK A expression may contribute to cancer cell survival through activities that enhance NF-kB, mTOR, Raf1, Myc, Wnt, or AKT signaling pathways [23]. Because AK A interacts with p53 at multiple levels, cancer cells with a deficient p53-p21$^{Waf1/Cip1}$ postmitotic checkpoint function may be more susceptible to AK inhibition [18, 24].

AK overexpression is also associated with a mitogenic phenotype and genetic instability [25, 26]. Resulting tumor cell non-diploidy contributes to uncontrolled cell cycle progression and promotes cell survival. These effects are synergistic with histone deacetylases in regulating cell proliferation and survival through activation of AKT/mTOR signaling in lymphomas [27]. AK C is overexpressed in several cancers and cancer cell lines, but its role in carcinogenesis and effect on tumor cell proliferation is unclear [28, 29]. Similar to AK B, overexpressed AK C binds to and localizes with the IAP protein survivin in mitotic cells [15, 27]. However, a clear role for AK C in tumorigenesis has not been identified.

2.2 Role of aurora kinases in drug resistance

Drug resistance remains a major challenge in oncology, regardless of whether cancer resistance to drug therapy is de novo and/or acquired. Elevated AK A and B expression is associated with chemoresistance in multiple tumor types and to different classes of anticancer drugs [30–39]. AK A has been implicated in the development of resistance and reduced sensitivity to microtubule-targeted chemotherapy [11, 31, 40–42]. Elevated levels override the spindle assembly checkpoint (SAC) responsible for monitoring defective mitotic spindle formation, thus conferring resistance to paclitaxel-induced apoptosis [42]. Similarly, there was a dose-dependent association between AK B expression in cell lines and resistance to paclitaxel [43]. AK activity also contributes to resistance to platinum-containing agents, and sensitivity to these drugs in vitro can be restored by AK inhibition [30, 38, 44]. These mechanisms present a potential opportunity to inhibit AK to restore or enhance drug sensitivity, which has been demonstrated preclinically [23]. This strategy holds implications for combination therapies with AK inhibitors and their potential role for relapsed/refractory malignancies including PTCL.

3. Aurora kinase inhibition in PTCL

Given the poor clinical outcomes associated with PTCL, more effective treatments informed by a better understanding of PTCL biology are needed. Several subtypes of PTCL have shown to overexpress AK A and B [45–47], making them an attractive therapeutic target. CD8+ T cells expressing STAT5BN642H, the most frequent STAT5B mutation found in patients with leukemias and lymphomas, were exquisitely sensitive to AK inhibition in a transgenic mouse model [48]. Given their role in multiple oncogenic processes, inhibition of AKs has a potential of halting malignant progression in PTCL.

Multiple preclinical and clinical studies have been conducted to explore the role of AK inhibitors in the treatment of advanced PTCL. Small molecules designed to bind competitively and reversibly to the ATP-binding pocket have been developed for all three AKs, including isoform-specific and pan-AK inhibitors [15, 21, 49]. AK isoform selectivity and inhibitory activity differ among individual agents. However, it is unclear whether a strategy of selective or pan-AK inhibition will provide superior efficacy [15, 19] without compromising safety.

3.1 Preclinical studies involving aurora kinase inhibitors

AK inhibitors were first studied in solid organ tumors and in hematologic tumor cell lines other than PTCL. Agents that have undergone preclinical evaluation in lymphomas are listed in **Table 1**. Much focus has been on AK A inhibition, as the mechanism of AK B in cancer is less clear.

Alisertib is a potent inhibitor of AK A, with a half maximal inhibitory concentration (IC_{50}) value of 1.2 nmol/L [50]. It has less activity against AK B, with an IC_{50} value of 396.5 nmol/L. Alisertib was studied in colorectal cancer and non-Hodgkin's lymphoma tumor cell lines in vivo and in vitro. In vitro, alisertib showed inhibition of proliferation in tumor cell lines, more so for lymphoma cell lines. In vivo, alisertib caused tumor growth inhibition (TGI) of 43.3, 84.2, and 94.7% when given at doses of 3, 10, and 30 mg/kg, respectively, in nude mice with subcutaneous colorectal HCT-116 cell. In a non-Hodgkin's lymphoma model ONI-LY19, there was tumor regression (TR) when alisertib was given at doses of 20 and 30 mg/kg [50]. Based on preliminary data from this study and similar preclinical studies of solid organ and hematological malignancies, phase I clinical trials involving alisertib in r/r PTCL were conducted.

The first preclinical study of alisertib involving PTCL cell lines was conducted by Qi et al. [47]. In this in vitro study, alisertib was tested on two mouse PTCL cell lines, TIB-48 and CRL-2396. AK A contributes to autophosphorylation on Thr288 in the activation loop. Alisertib at 0.1 μM completely inhibited AK A autophosphorylation on Thr288. Analysis of DNA content with flow cytometry showed that treatment of both PTCL cell lines with alisertib at 0.5, 1, and 1.5 μM resulted in cell cycle arrest in G2/M phase and there was evidence of endoreduplication resulting in

Name	Target (IC_{50} *in vitro*)	Sponsor	Comments
AT9283	Aurora A (3 nM) Aurora B (3 nM)	Astex	Multikinase inhibitor, including JAK2, JAK3, Abl T3151, Flt3
AZD1152 (barasertib)	Aurora A (1369) Aurora B (0.37 nM)	AstraZeneca	
Chiauranib	Aurora B (0.37 nM)	Chipscreen Biosciences	Multikinase inhibitor, including VEGFRs, c-KIT, and PDGFRs
MLN8237 (alisertib)	Aurora A (1.2 nM) Aurora B (396.5 nM)	Takeda/millennium Pharmaceuticals	Aurora A
TAK-901	Aurora A (21 nM) Aurora B (15 nM)	Takeda	Pan-Aurora

Table 1.
Aurora kinase inhibitors studied for lymphomas (from: Refs. [15, 20, 49, 60]).

polyploidy. These changes led to dose-dependent apoptosis of both cell lines when alisertib was used at 100 nM or higher.

Zullo et al. studied the cytotoxic effects of alisertib in vivo [51]. In addition, the effects of various combination drug regimens involving alisertib in vitro and in vivo on cell lines of r/r TCL were also studied. Alisertib alone showed concentration and strong time-dependent cytotoxicity with the lowest IC_{50} value achieved at 72 hours noted to be 60–1000 nm/L. Alisertib (IC_{10}–IC_{30}) given along with romidepsin (IC_{10}–IC_{20}) had a synergistic interaction in vitro in eight different TCL cell lines following 72 hours of drug exposure [51]. The greatest interaction was seen in C5MJ, an alisertib-resistant ATLL HTLV-1 Tax^+ cell line. This combination induced polyploidy in all TCL cell lines after 48 hours of treatment. There was also evidence of increased apoptosis with approximately 13 and 52% of cells showing apoptosis with increasing concentrations of alisertib (50 nmol/L and 100 nm/L) used. In this same trial, in vivo analysis with this combination regimen was conducted on a xenograft model using HH cell lines of TCL. The combination drug regimen was statistically superior compared to single agent alone and control group cohort (dimethyl sulfoxide) in decreasing the mean tumor burden over time ($p < 0.05$) and in prolonging the survival in mice ($p < 0.05$) by day 58. Drug concentration analysis in the animals inside the tumors showed that concentration of alisertib in the combination tumor samples increased at 1 (400 vs. 100 nmol/L) and 6 hours (300 vs. 150 nmol/L) compared to tumor samples in mice where drug was given alone. These data support synergistic cytotoxicity of a combination drug regimen of alisertib plus romidepsin [51]. In the same study, alisertib was also evaluated in combination with other drugs including pralatrexate or ixazomib, but there were no synergetic interactions in vitro in TCL cell lines.

Immunohistochemistry (IHC) analysis of tumor samples from patients treated with alisertib for r/r PTCL (SWOG 1108) showed a high Ki-67 and programmed death ligand (PD-L1): PD-1 staining ratio of 8.9-fold [52]. Increased levels of PD-L1 are associated with immune suppression. In view of this, Islam et al. conducted a study where alisertib was given along with PD-LI antibody (BE0101,

Bio X Cell, NH) in mice with r/r PTCL xenografts (CRL-2396 cells) [52]. Since the pan-PI3K inhibitor (PF-04691502) inhibits expression of the PD-L1 along with vincristine, these were also added to the former drug combination, and the results were compared between the two groups. Alisertib given alone resulted in tumor growth regression of ~30%, whereas PD-L1 antibody given alone had no anti-PTCL activity. Alisertib plus PD-L1 antibody resulted in ~90% TGI, but 20% of mice had a relapse at 2 weeks and 50% mice relapsed at 4 weeks. The combination of alisertib plus PD-L1 antibody plus pan-PI3K inhibitor and vincristine showed a 100% TGI. Only 25% of mice had recurrence at 4 weeks after discontinuation of treatment. It was noted that the OS with the four-drug regimen ($p < 0.0001$) was statistically superior to the two-drug combination.

3.2 Clinical trials involving aurora kinase inhibitors

AK A inhibitors have been studied in clinical trials after antitumor activity was shown in multiple in vitro and in vivo studies (**Table 2**). In two phase I trials by Cervantes et al. (n = 59) and Dees et al. (n = 87) in patients with advanced solid organ malignancies, the maximum tolerated dose of alisertib was 50 mg twice a day for 7 days in a 21-day cycle [53, 54]. Similarly, in another phase I study by Kelly et al. (n = 58), alisertib was evaluated in patients with multiple relapsed/refractory hematologic malignancies (multiple myeloma, non-Hodgkin's lymphoma and chronic lymphocytic leukemia) [55]. In this study there were two patients with advanced PTCL. Just as with the other phase I studies, this study also determined that the MTD for alisertib was 50 mg twice a day for 7 days. The drug pharmacokinetics was also studied, with the terminal elimination half-life noted to be 19.5 hours. The safety analysis showed that most frequent grade 3 or greater adverse effects were hematological in nature including neutropenia (45%), thrombocytopenia (28%), anemia (19%), and leukopenia (19%). One patient with PTCL experienced a PR.

Given the promising outcomes of alisertib in preclinical studies and previous phase I clinical trials, phase II trials were conducted for PTCL patients [56, 57]. In one such study by Friedberg et al. (n = 48), alisertib was given to patients with multiple hematological malignancies (diffuse large B-cell lymphoma, mantle cell lymphoma, transformed follicular lymphoma, Burkitt's lymphoma, non-cutaneous T-cell lymphoma) at a dose of 50 mg twice a day for 7 days in 21-day cycles. This study included eight patients with advanced PTCL. Four of eight patients (ORR = 50%) with advanced PTCL showed a clinical response (CR/PR). Three patients that showed response continued to be in remission and had received alisertib for greater than 1 year at the time of publication of the study [57]. In the phase II study by Barr et al. (n = 37) patients with various subtypes of r/r PTCL (PTAL, NOS (n = 13), AITL (n = 9), adult T-cell leukemia/lymphoma (n = 4), anaplastic large-cell lymphoma (n = 2), extra nodal natural killer/T-cell lymphoma (n = 2), and transformed mycosis fungoides (n = 7)) received alisertib at the RP2D. In patients with PTCL, the ORR was 30% (CR = 7%, PR = 23%). The long-term outcomes were reported for the whole group and not reported for PTCL subtypes. The median PFS time was noted to be 3 months with a 1-year PFS rate of 8%. The median OS was determined to be 8 months, with OS at 1 year estimated to be 30% for the entire group. The long-term outcomes in this study could have been negatively biased because none of patients with transformed mycosis fungoides showed any clinical response with alisertib. As seen in the phase I studies, the most common grade 3 or higher adverse effects were due to myelosuppression (neutropenia 32%, anemia 30%, thrombocytopenia 24%). Common non-hematologic adverse effects included fatigue (50%), alopecia (24%), and mucositis (20%) [56].

Author	Phase	No. of patients	MTD	Response	EFS/PFS	OS	SE (>grade 3)
Kelly et al. [55]	I	2	50 mg bid for 7 days	PR = 50%	NL	NL	Neutropenia = 9% Gi side affects Alopecia
Friedberg et al. [57]	II	8	NR	ORR = 50%	1 yr. = 75%	1 yr. = 75%	Neutropenia = 63% Leukemia = 54% Anemia = 35% Thrombocytopenia = 33% Stomatitis = 15% Fatigue = 6%
Barr et al. [56]	II	30	NR	ORR = 30% CR = 7% PR = 23%	NLS	NLS	Neutropenia = 32% Anemia = 30% Thrombocytopenia = 24%
O'Connor et al. [58]	III	A = 120 C = 118	NR	ORR A = 33% ORR C = 43%	mPFS A = 3.7 m mPFS M = 3.4 m	mOS A = 9.9 m mOS M = 12.2 m	Grade 3 A ≥ 85% Grade 3 M ≥ 81%

Abbreviations: No., number; MTD, maximum tolerated dose; NR, not reached; PR, partial remission; ORR, overall response rate; CR, complete remission; EFS, event free survival; PFS, progression-free survival; SE, side effects; NL, not listed; NLS, not listed separately for alisertib; mPFS, median progression-free survival; mOS, median overall survival; A, alisertib; M, monotherapy; SE(>grade 3), greater than grade 3 side effects; yr. = year.

Table 2.
Clinical trials of alisertib in treatment of relapsed/refractory PTCL.

Based on good tolerance and positive response/survival seen in patients with advanced PTCL in multiple phase I and II studies with alisertib, an international phase III randomized controlled study was conducted [58]. In this study, patients with r/r PTCL received either enteric-coated alisertib (n = 120) at a dose of 50 mg twice a day for 7 days in a 21-day cycle or investigator's choice of monotherapy treatment (n = 118) using pralatrexate, romidepsin, or gemcitabine. The treatment was intended to be continued until disease progression, unacceptable toxicity, or for 2 years. An interim analysis showed that ORR, median PFS, and median OS were 33%, 3.7 months, and 9.9 months versus 43%, 3.3 months, and 12.2 months, respectively, with alisertib and investigator's choice of treatment. The rate of grade 3 or higher side effects was 85% for alisertib and 81% for the investigator's treatment choice. Since the interim analysis of this phase III study failed to show superior outcomes of alisertib compared to investigator's preferred choice of drugs, a decision was made by the investigators to discontinue the study.

Given the promise of combination regimen with alisertib given along with another drug that is generally used for patients with r/r PTCL in preclinical studies, phase I clinical studies with some of these regimens are in progress. In one such phase I study by Strati et al., alisertib plus romidepsin in patients with PTCL (n = 3) or aggressive B-cell lymphoma (n = 16) [59] showed that the drug combination was well tolerated with most common grade 3–4 side effects due to myelosuppression. One patient with PTCL showed a CR and other two patients showed stable disease. The enrollment for the highest dose for these regimens is ongoing. Similarly, in another phase I study, vorinostat plus alisertib is being evaluated for patients with r/r PTCL (NCT01567709).

4. Conclusion and future directions

PTCLs are highly aggressive clinically challenging diseases, with high rates of relapse, and poor overall survival with traditional cell cycle directed anti-lymphoma therapies. Effective treatment options are limited for patients with newly diagnosed and r/r PTCL. AKs are aberrantly expressed and active in PTCL, leading to uncontrolled cell division, immune suppression, and oncogenesis. AK inhibition leads to catastrophic errors of mitosis, such as defective cytokinesis, misaligned centrosomes, and mitotic spindle malformation, culminating in apoptosis [60, 61]. However, drug-resistant non-diploid cells can enter the cell cycle by reductive divisions during intermittent therapy [62]. Several AK inhibitors have been studied preclinically and clinically in trials for patients with r/r PTCL. Despite showing benefit in phase II studies, an interim analysis of a phase III trial of alisertib, a selective AK inhibitor, failed to show improved response or survival rates compared to standard of care single-agent monotherapy for patients with r/r PTCL. However, targeting cell proliferation plus immune suppression in preclinical studies of novel combinations of alisertib plus a PD-L1 inhibitor plus a pan-PIK3 inhibitor plus vincristine as well as combined HDAC inhibition plus alisertib shows synergistic activity and prolonged survival in mouse models of PTCL. Furthermore, AK inhibition may improve or restore tumor sensitivity to anticancer agents, particularly microtubule-targeted and platinum-containing drugs in the context of pathogenic *TP53* mutant status. Continued clinical studies of novel drug combinations with AK inhibitors are warranted to target not only malignant T cells but also their immune suppressive T cells residing in the tumor microenvironment.

Acknowledgements

We acknowledge funding from the SWOG/Hope Foundation Impact Award to DM.

Conflict of interest

There is no conflict of interest for all three authors.

Author details

Pavan Tenneti[1], Lisa E. Davis[2] and Daruka Mahadevan[3]*

1 Banner Estrella Medical Center, Phoenix, AZ, USA

2 College of Pharmacy, University of Arizona, Tucson, AZ, USA

3 University of Arizona Cancer Center, Tucson, AZ, USA

*Address all correspondence to: dmahadevan@uacc.arizona.edu

References

[1] The non-Hodgkin's Lymphoma classification project. A clinical evaluation of the International Lymphoma Study Group classification of non-Hodgkin's lymphoma. Blood. 1997;**89**(11):3909-3918

[2] Cutucache CE, Herek TA. Burrowing through the heterogeneity: Review of mouse models of PTCL-NOS. Frontiers in Oncology. 2016;**6**:206

[3] Vose J, Armitage J, Weisenburger D. International peripheral T-cell and natural killer/T-cell lymphoma study: Pathology findings and clinical outcomes. Journal of Clinical Oncology. 2008;**26**(25):4124-4130

[4] Mahadevan D et al. Phase 2 trial of combined cisplatin, etoposide, gemcitabine, and methylprednisolone (PEGS) in peripheral T-cell non-Hodgkin lymphoma: Southwest Oncology Group Study S0350. Cancer. 2013;**119**(2):371-379

[5] Fanale MA et al. Five-year outcomes for frontline brentuximab vedotin with CHP for CD30-expressing peripheral T-cell lymphomas. Blood. 2018;**131**(19):2120-2124

[6] d'Amore F et al. Up-front autologous stem-cell transplantation in peripheral T-cell lymphoma: NLG-T-01. Journal of Clinical Oncology. 2012;**30**(25):3093-3099

[7] T-Cell Lymphomas. MS-21 & MS-22. National Comprehensive Cancer Network Guidelines; 2018. Available from: https://www.nccn.org/professionals/physician_gls/pdf/t-cell.pdf [Accessed: May 21, 2018]

[8] Broccoli A, Argnani L, Zinzani PL. Peripheral T-cell lymphomas: Focusing on novel agents in relapsed and refractory disease. Cancer Treatment Reviews. 2017;**60**:120-129

[9] Carmena M, Earnshaw WC. The cellular geography of aurora kinases. Nature Reviews. Molecular Cell Biology. 2003;**4**(11):842-854

[10] Ducat D, Zheng Y. Aurora kinases in spindle assembly and chromosome segregation. Experimental Cell Research. 2004;**301**(1):60-67

[11] Marumoto T, Zhang D, Saya H. Aurora-A—A guardian of poles. Nature Reviews Cancer. 2005;**5**(1):42-50

[12] Fu J et al. Roles of aurora kinases in mitosis and tumorigenesis. Molecular Cancer Research. 2007;**5**(1):1-10

[13] Zhang X. Aurora kinases. Current Biology. 2008;**18**(4):R146-R148

[14] Goldenson B, Crispino JD. The aurora kinases in cell cycle and leukemia. Oncogene. 2015;**34**(5):537-545

[15] Borisa AC, Bhatt HG. A comprehensive review on Aurora kinase: Small molecule inhibitors and clinical trial studies. European Journal of Medicinal Chemistry. 2017;**140**:1-19

[16] Afonso O, Figueiredo AC, Maiato H. Late mitotic functions of Aurora kinases. Chromosoma. 2017;**126**(1):93-103

[17] Karthigeyan D et al. Biology of Aurora A kinase: Implications in cancer manifestation and therapy. Medicinal Research Reviews. 2011;**31**(5):757-793

[18] Hilton JF, Shapiro GI. Aurora kinase inhibition as an anticancer strategy. Journal of Clinical Oncology. 2014;**32**(1):57-59

[19] Green MR, Woolery JE, Mahadevan D. Update on Aurora kinase targeted therapeutics in oncology. Expert Opinion on Drug Discovery. 2011;**6**(3):291-307

[20] Gautschi O et al. Aurora kinases as anticancer drug targets. Clinical Cancer Research. 2008;**14**(6):1639-1648

[21] Bavetsias V, Linardopoulos S. Aurora kinase inhibitors: Current status and outlook. Frontiers in Oncology. 2015;**5**:278

[22] Slattery SD et al. Aurora-C kinase supports mitotic progression in the absence of Aurora-B. Cell Cycle. 2009;**8**(18):2984-2994

[23] Tang A et al. Aurora kinases: Novel therapy targets in cancers. Oncotarget. 2017;**8**(14):23937-23954

[24] Ujhazy P, Stewart D. DNA repair. Journal of Thoracic Oncology. 2009;**4**(11 Suppl 3):S1068-S1070

[25] Keen N, Taylor S. Mitotic drivers—Inhibitors of the Aurora B kinase. Cancer Metastasis Reviews. 2009;**28**(1-2):185-195

[26] Smith SL et al. Overexpression of aurora B kinase (AURKB) in primary non-small cell lung carcinoma is frequent, generally driven from one allele, and correlates with the level of genetic instability. British Journal of Cancer. 2005;**93**(6):719-729

[27] Wang C et al. Aurora-B and HDAC synergistically regulate survival and proliferation of lymphoma cell via AKT, mTOR and Notch pathways. European Journal of Pharmacology. 2016;**779**:1-7

[28] Kobayashi M et al. Analysis of Aurora kinase expressions and cell cycle regulation by Aurora-C in leukemia cells. In: American Society of Hematology Annual Conference (ASH '06). Blood. 2006;**108**(11):1366-1366

[29] Kimura M et al. Cell cycle-dependent expression and centrosome localization of a third human aurora/Ipl1-related protein kinase, AIK3. The Journal of Biological Chemistry. 1999;**274**(11):7334-7340

[30] Akiyama M et al. Hypersensitivity to aurora kinase inhibitors in cells resistant against platinum-containing anticancer agents. Anti-Cancer Agents in Medicinal Chemistry. 2014;**14**(7):1042-1050

[31] Cirak Y et al. Aurora A overexpression in breast cancer patients induces taxane resistance and results in worse prognosis. Journal of BUON. 2015;**20**(6):1414-1419

[32] Hole S et al. Aurora kinase A and B as new treatment targets in aromatase inhibitor-resistant breast cancer cells. Breast Cancer Research and Treatment. 2015;**149**(3):715-726

[33] Katsha A et al. Activation of EIF4E by Aurora kinase A depicts a novel druggable axis in everolimus-resistant cancer cells. Clinical Cancer Research. 2017;**23**(14):3756-3768

[34] Li Y et al. Silencing Aurora A leads to re-sensitization of breast cancer cells to taxol through downregulation of SRC-mediated ERK and mTOR pathways. Oncology Reports. 2017;**38**(4):2011-2022

[35] Long ZJ et al. A novel compound against oncogenic Aurora kinase A overcomes imatinib resistance in chronic myeloid leukemia cells. International Journal of Oncology. 2015;**46**(6):2488-2496

[36] Xu J et al. Aurora-A contributes to cisplatin resistance and lymphatic metastasis in non-small cell lung cancer and predicts poor prognosis. Journal of Translational Medicine. 2014;**12**:200

[37] Zhang Y et al. Elevated Aurora B expression contributes to chemoresistance and poor prognosis in breast cancer. International Journal of Clinical and Experimental Pathology. 2015;**8**(1):751-757

[38] Zhu Q et al. Inhibition of Aurora A kinase by alisertib induces

autophagy and cell cycle arrest and increases chemosensitivity in human hepatocellular carcinoma HepG2 cells. Current Cancer Drug Targets. 2017;**17**(4):386-401

[39] Kollareddy M et al. Aurora kinase inhibitors: Progress towards the clinic. Investigational New Drugs. 2012;**30**(6):2411-2432

[40] Nishida N et al. High copy amplification of the Aurora-A gene is associated with chromosomal instability phenotype in human colorectal cancers. Cancer Biology & Therapy. 2007;**6**(4):525-533

[41] Gritsko TM et al. Activation and overexpression of centrosome kinase BTAK/Aurora-A in human ovarian cancer. Clinical Cancer Research. 2003;**9**(4):1420-1426

[42] Anand S, Penrhyn-Lowe S, Venkitaraman AR. AURORA-A amplification overrides the mitotic spindle assembly checkpoint, inducing resistance to Taxol. Cancer Cell. 2003;**3**(1):51-62

[43] Al-Khafaji AS et al. Aurora B expression modulates paclitaxel response in non-small cell lung cancer. British Journal of Cancer. 2017;**116**(5):592-599

[44] Wang L et al. Cisplatin-resistant cancer cells are sensitive to Aurora kinase A inhibition by alisertib. Molecular Oncology. 2017;**11**(8):981-995

[45] Mahadevan D et al. Transcript profiling in peripheral T-cell lymphoma, not otherwise specified, and diffuse large B-cell lymphoma identifies distinct tumor profile signatures. Molecular Cancer Therapeutics. 2005;**4**(12):1867-1879

[46] Kanagal-Shamanna R et al. Differential expression of aurora-A kinase in T-cell lymphomas. Modern Pathology. 2013;**26**(5):640-647

[47] Qi W et al. Alisertib (MLN8237) an investigational agent suppresses Aurora A and B activity, inhibits proliferation, promotes endo-reduplication and induces apoptosis in T-NHL cell lines supporting its importance in PTCL treatment. Leukemia Research. 2013;**37**(4):434-439

[48] Pham HTT et al. STAT5BN642H is a driver mutation for T cell neoplasia. The Journal of Clinical Investigation. 2018;**128**(1):387-401

[49] Kitzen JJ, de Jonge MJ, Verweij J. Aurora kinase inhibitors. Critical Reviews in Oncology/Hematology. 2010;**73**(2):99-110

[50] Manfredi MG et al. Characterization of alisertib (MLN8237), an investigational small-molecule inhibitor of aurora A kinase using novel in vivo pharmacodynamic assays. Clinical Cancer Research. 2011;**17**(24):7614-7624

[51] Zullo KM et al. Aurora A kinase inhibition selectively synergizes with histone deacetylase inhibitor through cytokinesis failure in T-cell lymphoma. Clinical Cancer Research. 2015;**21**(18):4097-4109

[52] Islam S et al. Co-targeting aurora kinase with PD-L1 and PI3K abrogates immune checkpoint mediated proliferation in peripheral T-cell lymphoma: A novel therapeutic strategy. Oncotarget. 2017;**8**(59):100326-100338

[53] Cervantes A et al. Phase I pharmacokinetic/pharmacodynamic study of MLN8237, an investigational, oral, selective aurora a kinase inhibitor, in patients with advanced solid tumors. Clinical Cancer Research. 2012;**18**(17):4764-4774

[54] Dees EC et al. Phase I study of aurora A kinase inhibitor MLN8237 in

advanced solid tumors: Safety, pharmacokinetics, pharmacodynamics, and bioavailability of two oral formulations. Clinical Cancer Research. 2012;**18**(17):4775-4784

[55] Kelly KR et al. Phase I study of MLN8237--investigational Aurora A kinase inhibitor--in relapsed/refractory multiple myeloma, non-Hodgkin lymphoma and chronic lymphocytic leukemia. Investigational New Drugs. 2014;**32**(3):489-499

[56] Barr PM et al. Phase II intergroup trial of alisertib in relapsed and refractory peripheral T-cell lymphoma and transformed mycosis fungoides: SWOG 1108. Journal of Clinical Oncology. 2015;**33**(21):2399-2404

[57] Friedberg JW et al. Phase II study of alisertib, a selective Aurora A kinase inhibitor, in relapsed and refractory aggressive B- and T-cell non-Hodgkin lymphomas. Journal of Clinical Oncology. 2014;**32**(1):44-50

[58] O'Connor OA et al. First multicenter, randomized phase 3 study in patients (Pts) with relapsed/refractory (R/R) peripheral T-cell lymphoma (PTCL): Alisertib (MLN8237) versus investigator's choice. In: 57th American Soceity of Hematology Annual Meeting and Exposition (ASH '15); 5-8 December 2015. Blood. 2015;**126**(23):341-341

[59] Strati P et al. A phase 1 trial of alisertib and romidepsin for relapsed/refractory aggressive B-cell and T-cell lymphomas. In: 59th American Society of Hematology and Oncology Annual Meeting and Expedition(ASH '17); 9-12 December 2017. Blood. 2017;**130** (Suppl 1):4074-4074

[60] Carvajal RD, Tse A, Schwartz GK. Aurora kinases: New targets for cancer therapy. Clinical Cancer Research. 2006;**12**(23):6869-6875

[61] Girdler F et al. Validating Aurora B as an anti-cancer drug target. Journal of Cell Science. 2006;**119**(Pt 17):3664-3675

[62] Islam S et al. Disruption of aneuploidy and senescence induced by Aurora inhibition promotes intrinsic apoptosis in double hit or double expressor diffuse large B-cell lymphomas. Molecular Cancer Therapeutics. 2017;**16**(10):2083-2093

[63] Mahadevan D, Vick E, Huber B, Morales C, Cooke L, Spier CM, et al. Blood. Aurora Plus PI3K Inhibition Abrogates PD-L1 Induction in Peripheral T-Cell Non-Hodgkin Lymphoma. 2015;**126**:1560